LIFESTYLE PRESCRIPTION FOR DIABETES AND PREDIABETES

5C LIFESTYLE PROGRAM
TREAT THE CAUSE, NOT JUST THE SYMPTOMS

DR. AMENA SADIYA, Ph.D
(Nutritionist)

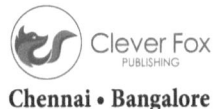

Chennai • Bangalore

CLEVER FOX PUBLISHING
Chennai, India

Published by CLEVER FOX PUBLISHING 2023
Copyright © Dr. Amena Sadiya Ph.D 2023

All Rights Reserved.
ISBN: 978-93-56485-02-0

This book has been published with all reasonable efforts taken to make the material error-free after the consent of the author. No part of this book shall be used, reproduced in any manner whatsoever without written permission from the author, except in the case of brief quotations embodied in critical articles and reviews.

The Author of this book is solely responsible and liable for its content including but not limited to the views, representations, descriptions, statements, information, opinions and references ["Content"]. The Content of this book shall not constitute or be construed or deemed to reflect the opinion or expression of the Publisher or Editor. Neither the Publisher nor Editor endorse or approve the Content of this book or guarantee the reliability, accuracy or completeness of the Content published herein and do not make any representations or warranties of any kind, express or implied, including but not limited to the implied warranties of merchantability, fitness for a particular purpose. The Publisher and Editor shall not be liable whatsoever for any errors, omissions, whether such errors or omissions result from negligence, accident, or any other cause or claims for loss or damages of any kind, including without limitation, indirect or consequential loss or damage arising out of use, inability to use, or about the reliability, accuracy or sufficiency of the information contained in this book.

Illustrations by Samiya Zahra

"To all those who have inspired me to give back more than I receive and make a positive impact in the community by utilizing my skills and knowledge, I am deeply grateful."

ACKNOWLEDGEMENTS

*F*irst and foremost, I would like to praise and thank God, the almighty Allah, who has granted countless blessings, knowledge, and opportunities to me, so that I have been finally able to finish this book.

This book is, in many ways, a work of synthesis, built on a foundation of research, clinical experience and interaction with my patients and colleagues. Living and working in the United Arab Emirates for 18 years has given me the opportunity to work with many different nationalities, cultures, and regions that bring their own eating habits and choices to the table.

I have gained a profound understanding of how food is similar and different at the same time around the world. Despite the differences in food, the relationship between food and eating behaviours remains the same. I would like to take this opportunity to thank this multicultural and multinational community for its contribution to my knowledge and wisdom.

My education and training have made me a nutritionist and researcher. However, my parents, Tanveer Fatima and Gulam Samdani, have made me the person I am today. I thank them for instilling a dreamer in me.

Acknowledgements

I would like to thank my dear husband, Syed Fasi, for his unwavering support and patience. Being relentlessly supportive, believing in me, listening, critiquing, and pushing me forward throughout.

I cannot express my gratitude enough to my daughter, Samiya Zahra, a gifted artist and illustrator, who, at the age of 16, has been instrumental in providing illustrations and designing my book. It is your endless happiness and pleasure that I receive every day that makes me so happy.

I'd like to thank my brother, Dr. Imad Ali, for inspiring and motivating me to put together this book.

It has been Carole Fossey's exceptional expertise, keen eye for detail, and unwavering dedication have helped shape this book to its full potential. Her invaluable editing contribution enabled this book to reach its full potential. Thank you, Carole, for your unwavering commitment to excellence.

I would like to extend my heartfelt appreciation to Dr. Martin Carlsson for his invaluable role as a reviewer for this book. Dr. Carlsson's expertise and dedication have greatly enhanced the quality and credibility of this work.

I would like to express my sincere gratitude to Dr. Yohannes Tesfa for his unwavering support, encouragement, and invaluable feedback during the development of this book.

I would also like to thank my adorable and adorable bunnies, Cinnamon and Kaju, for always keeping me company and giving me much-needed relaxation time.

CONTENTS

Chapter 1 Introduction 1
Chapter 2 Insulin Resistance, Prediabetes and Diabetes.......... 18
Chapter 3 Carbs and Fat Metabolism – and Why
They Matter! 49
Chapter 4 Consequences of Diabetes: Heart, Nerves,
Eyes, and Kidneys... 90

The 5C program

Chapter 5 The 1st C — Condition Your Mind..................... 111
Chapter 6 The 2nd C - Choose, Cook, and Eat Real Food.... 143
Chapter 7 The 3rd C - Create Your Own Meal Plan 174
Chapter 8 The 4th C – Count on Active Movement,
Sound Sleep, and Stress management 231
Chapter 9 The 5th C- Capitalise on Technology 268

Appendix I *284*
Appendix II *291*
Appendix III *297*
References *307*
Index *330*

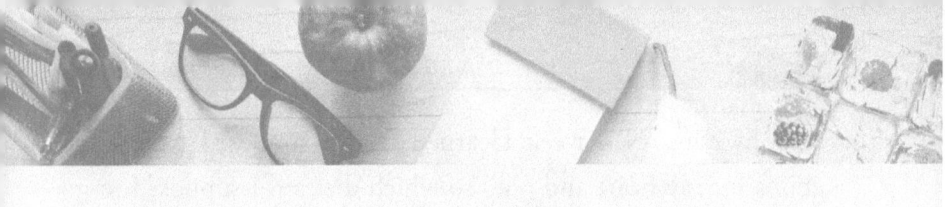

CHAPTER 1

INTRODUCTION

*I*f you are reading this book, then I am guessing you are looking for information and/or a solution for a health-related problem. If you are looking for a light at the end of the tunnel, you have found it!

In over 18 years of experience engaging with people with diabetes, prediabetes, weight gain, hypertension, cardiovascular diseases, or polycystic ovary syndrome, I have encountered many individuals who have succeeded in changing their health for good, as well as those who don't believe they can change themselves for the better, and those who are unsure what to do.

Perhaps something below may resonate with you:

"My doctor told me that I needed to control my blood glucose and take medications regularly. Despite taking all my medications regularly, my blood glucose and blood pressure seem to fluctuate into the higher range. As my mother did, I am worried that I will suffer from heart or eye problems."

"It's difficult to make sense of all the conflicting advice out there, and it's hard to figure out what's reliable and what's not. One day, they tell me to avoid grains because they're high in carbohydrates. Next week, I learned that I'm supposed to consume grains for my heart and gut. So which diet am I supposed to go with? Low-carbohydrate, low-fat, ketogenic or plant-based? Or just intermittent fasting? Every day, I hear something new. I have no faith in these diets."

"I'm busy. Really busy. I'm always working and taking care of my family. There's too much to do and there's never enough time. Can't cook meals, can't go out to exercise, can't sleep early. Sometimes I wonder, can I prevent my kids from these medical situations? I never want them to experience this. Can I do something to prevent them from developing these conditions?"

"This is my first pregnancy and my blood glucose levels have spiked. I've been careful throughout, despite being told I had to eat for two, I never indulged in sweets. Then why did I develop diabetes during my pregnancy? I'm worried sick about my unborn child. Will my child develop diabetes?"

"I've started a new diet for the third time this year. I know I'm overweight, and I really want to change. I constantly check social media and follow many influencers to stay up to date with diabetes. I set my goals, I listen to motivational speakers and start a regime, brimming with ambition. After a few weeks, I fizzle. I just can't cope with the daily routine and feel like this is not for me."

These are real issues and painful problems that people with diabetes, prediabetes or a metabolic condition face every day. Perhaps you too are facing an uncertain future after a diagnosis, or maybe you have been struggling for a long time trying to manage your existing condition and feeling powerless or confused by conflicting advice.

So where do you want to be instead?

Imagine waking up in the morning comfortable about the day ahead, feeling healthy and with enough energy to manage the day. Picture being able to maintain a weight that is healthy for you, easily and without having to struggle. Envisage a time where you will be setting the example for your children that you want to, and are secure in the knowledge that they will face their future with their health firmly in their own hands. Visualise the surprise on your doctor's face when they realise that you have reversed your condition and put yourself back into optimal health.

So, how are you going to get from where you are now to where you want to be? I believe it comes down to a simple formula for health, which has 3 simple but essential criteria.

1. The Will to Change
2. Taking Knowledge-Based Action
3. Giving Yourself Permission to Fail, and Bounce Back

Everything starts with your desire to change, seeking knowledge based on facts and not fads and tales. Since you have picked up this book, I believe that you have a desire to change and if that desire translates into action, then this book can be your key to manifesting your best self.

Most people have heard of Diabetes. But what do you really know about it? A diagnosis of diabetes can have a profound impact on a person and is a serious threat to life and also to your way of life. Managing diabetes requires significant changes to your daily routine. Most people are not ready for this.

There are extra medical appointments, information that you may not understand, and things you need to keep track of (glucose levels, medications). Your daily schedule is upended and you can feel at the mercy of something (the diagnosis) or someone (the medical professionals) which are out of your control. These changes can be emotionally, socially, and financially draining, leaving you feeling exhausted.

It doesn't have to be this way. You don't have to be a passive patient and allow diabetes to take control of your life; instead, you can take control and make it fit in with you. I often tell my patients, "There is nothing that a person with diabetes should do that a healthy person could ignore." In fact, the lifestyle recommendations for a healthy person or a diabetic person are more or less the same. The only difference is that a person with diabetes needs to pay immediate attention, or else it will have detrimental consequences. However, healthy people who continue to make bad choices will likely end up with these problems later on.

To enjoy life to the fullest, everyone needs to eat right, exercise more, cope with stress, and sleep well. Many people live their life as if these choices are optional until diabetes compels the need for the right lifestyle choices.

It is, therefore, important that you have definitive guidance about the following:

- How to distinguish between right and wrong information

- How to implement the appropriate changes
- How to adapt to the changes
- How to create new habits, that stick

The chances are that you will fall behind at times and that is absolutely ok. You are human, not a computer. We make mistakes! The trick lies in getting up and catching up again. And here's the good news:

Diabetes will no longer need to dominate your life. By putting yourself first and dealing with diabetes head-on, you and not your condition, will be in control.

You Are Not Alone, and That Is Scary!

Type 2 Diabetes is one of the fastest-growing lifestyle-induced (caused by poor lifestyle choices) diseases around the globe; it is perhaps the most notorious of all the diseases. In 2000, about 4.6% of the world population was diagnosed with diabetes. The number of people with diabetes nearly doubled to 9.8% by 2021, despite the growth spurt in medical research, technology, communication, and health awareness.[1]

As of the latest data provided by the International Diabetes Federation (IDF), one in ten adults around the world are living with diabetes. It is interesting to note that 2 out of 3 people with diabetes live in urban areas.[1] If you live in a city, take a moment to consider that one in six adults in your city lives with diabetes. This is a clear demonstration of the impact lifestyle choices have on the incidence of this disease. These are staggering statistics and all nations are guilty of not doing enough to bring down the size or struggles of the growing diabetic community.

The Roadblocks You Will Encounter

The quest to get healthy, feel energetic, and live life to the fullest is a one that millions of people embark on every year. There are a number of obstacles to achieving this goal, among them is inadequate and misleading information, the lack of tools that can be used to change deeply ingrained habits, and the difficulty in sustaining those changes.

Nowadays, you have access to a vast amount of information. The internet has revolutionised the way people access health information and make dietary choices. However, it can be difficult to distinguish between what is trustworthy and harmful information online. The amount of information is overwhelming, and the challenge is to identify reliable scientific information within the excessive noise of irrelevant, incorrect or even harmful information.

And how do you go about integrating that information into your daily decisions? What is right for you may not be appropriate for your friend. For instance, how many calories you need or your blood glucose target. The answer can differ from person to person.

After the Roadblocks – There is Sunshine

The general belief is that if you are diagnosed with diabetes or prediabetes, your fight is already lost. Sooner or later, they say you will gain weight, feel less energetic, spend your savings on medical expenses, incur inevitable diabetes complications, and may even suffer from a shorter lifespan.

Thankfully, this is not the only truth; however, it _is_ the truth if you do not take control of your diagnosis. All the potential threats stated above are avoidable or delayable if you make the right choices; I will be discussing them in further chapters.

Diabetes is categorised as a chronic disease, which means "persisting for a long time or recurring frequently." I believe this is because lifestyle choices made over the years have become chronic, i.e., they "persist for a long time and often recur when you fall back into poor habits."

Today, enough scientific evidence indicates that positive lifestyle changes can not only slow down the path toward ill health but also reverse that path. Provided you hold the steering wheel and firmly drive toward health and happiness rather than allow diabetes to lead your path to pain and despair.

Time to Empower Yourself

Unfortunately, many physicians are unaware of the powerful effect lifestyle changes can have on the prevention, management, and reversal of diabetes. The absence of training, difficulty enforcing behavioural changes, insufficient resources, lack of time, non-compliance of the patient, or other factors may contribute to this ignorance.

There have been many ad-hoc initiatives to counsel people with diabetes, which have led to failure. That's because one size does not fit all, and more personalised and individualised approaches are required in order to achieve success in diabetes counseling.

If I was being cynical, I could point out that there is no money to be made by pharmaceutical companies from healthy eating. Fruit and vegetables cannot be patented. And we live in a system which seeks to treat and discover new medicines, not one that focuses on prevention.

It is unfortunate that our healthcare system only treats symptoms like high blood glucose, high blood pressure, or high blood lipid levels but does not address the causes of these symptoms, such as unhealthy diet, inactivity, weight gain, insulin resistance, stress, or poor sleeping patterns; which contribute to and often cause these symptoms.

The health services cover the pills and procedures prescribed by doctors, but not the time spent empowering the patient with information about the benefits and importance of leading healthy lifestyles. As long as we are rewarded and reimbursed for treating symptoms, I do not expect great changes in medical care around lifestyle-induced diseases.

In my fire safety training, I was taught that the first step in putting out a fire is to remove the source of fuel. As an analogy, fighting diabetes is very similar to firefighting. You develop diabetes as a result of a state of inflammation (the fire) within your body, and the fuel for this inflammation includes an unhealthy diet, inactivity, poor sleeping patterns, and mental stress.

The medications you get will serve as extinguishers to put out the fire temporarily. However, as long as the source of fuel is not removed, only half the work is done, and it will reoccur.

Typically, a routine clinic visit involves blood tests and medication prescriptions to slow down the inevitable deterioration of diabetes complications. It does nothing to extinguish the fuel of diabetes.

I do not seek to undermine the importance and role of physicians and medications in the management of diabetes. The value of millennia of medical research, experimentation, knowledge, and practice is not something I would ever tar or malign.

Nevertheless, I would like to draw your attention to the elephant in the room—the complete picture. Rather than concentrating primarily on symptoms, we must work equally to find the underlying causes of these symptoms.

As long as we operate in a money-driven healthcare model, disease prevention and the role of lifestyle will be faulty and fragmented.

My Aspiration

Over the last two decades, I have worked as a nutritionist, lifestyle medicine professional, and researcher with people with diabetes and lifestyle diseases. Over these years, I have learned that there is a lot of inadequate and false information going around. I strongly believe that this false information needs to be erased before the real truth is revealed, as it is a truth that is too beautiful to be hidden any longer.

To take charge of your health you need to first "undo before you do." The journey toward robust health will be effective if you take a few steps backward and undo a lot of false information, beliefs, ideas, and their effects on you before you acquire sound knowledge.

It is essential that you combine precise scientific information with the most recent research evidence, take steps to change your behaviour, and use some simple tools to facilitate these changes. The combination of all the above is what will effect lasting change on your health and wellbeing.

When I started working on this book two years ago, I decided it would be most effective to empower individuals directly with information and tools to manage their own lifestyle to improve their diabetes. This does not undermine the importance of healthcare providers but simply helps you to sit in the driver's seat and steer toward health responsibly.

This book will provide you with self-help techniques so that you are able to develop a healthy relationship with diabetes rather than an uneasy relationship

What does this book offer?

Throughout this book, I will discuss how your body is wrecked by insulin resistance, leading to prediabetes and diabetes, and how your food can either harm or heal your body.

I will also discuss how you can achieve your health goals by becoming your own master, which is essential in order to manage your diabetes.

Your progress will make you feel great, look amazing, and reduce the risk of long-term complications of diabetes like coronary artery disease, neuropathy, nephropathy, cancer, chronic kidney disease, fatty liver, and Alzheimer's disease.

This book will also teach you about the physiological changes associated with prediabetes and diabetes, the interpretation of basic blood tests, and how medications are used to control blood glucose.

Due to the enormous impact of diet on blood glucose, I will discuss in great detail the basics of food, the role of nutrients, and various dietary patterns based on the latest scientific literature—the scientist in me cannot ignore this.

Everything in this book is supported by scientific research and referenced for your further reading. However, I have tried to explain the scientific evidence in simple terms to help you better understand the "hows" and "whys."

Glucose is the major source of energy for your body, and your blood maintains an optimum level at all times. However, the presence of disproportionate glucose levels in the blood for a long time causes damage and diabetes.

Type 1 and 2 diabetes are two distinct conditions caused by different factors, hence, managed differently. Other rare types of diabetes are also discussed in later chapters. The common factor in all types is that the blood sugar level in people's blood is too high; this condition is known as hyperglycemia.

In patients with diabetes of any type, once hyperglycemia occurs, they are at risk for developing the same chronic complications, though their rates of progression may differ.

The purpose of this book is to assist you in achieving long-term, sustainable lifestyle changes that will result in effective control of blood glucose, blood pressure, blood lipid, and weight. By following the simple strategies presented in the 5C Lifestyle Prescriptions, you can reduce or even eliminate your medications as well.

5C Lifestyle Prescription to Prevent, Control or Reverse Diabetes

It has been my privilege to engage with thousands of people over time, helping them manage their diabetes. Through reading several research articles, conducting research studies to examine the impact of lifestyle interventions, and publishing research papers on nutrition, lifestyle, and diabetes, I have developed a roadmap to help you understand how to manage your lifestyle on your own.

This is what I call a 5C Lifestyle Prescription since it includes five fundamental components:-

Component 1C: Condition Your Mind

The mind is the source of all change, so conditioning your mind will prepare you for any major life changes that you want to make. By doing so, you will be prepared to take on any challenge and overcome any obstacle that may arise. This component will help you modify your thoughts, attitudes, thinking patterns, and beliefs related to eating, moving, and sleeping in order to create a physical change.

Once you start to connect your lifestyle choices with your body and mind, you will experience harmony and reap the rewards. Your choices will no longer revolve around something you should do but rather around something you want to do. Eventually, it becomes your way of life, which is what I call powerful medicine.

Component 2C: Choose, Cook and Eat Real Food

Are you eating real food? To know the answer to this you must ask, what is real food?

Real food will be close to its natural form and minimally processed with no added chemicals or preservatives; it is all about preserving healthy nutrients in their natural form.

Next time you're at the supermarket, take a closer look at the items in your cart and consider how many of the food items are close to their natural state. Think about how many of these items you had access to as a child and how many your parents had access to as a child. For instance, did they have access to nuggets, frozen pizza, energy drinks, instant noodles, or flavoured milk; the answer is NO!

After learning how to identify and choose real food, you must consume it over anything else, for good health. In the last 50 years, the daily calorie consumption by the average person has gone up from nearly 2200 kcal to 2800 kcal (+500 kcal) globally.[2] So has the prevalence of lifestyle diseases and diabetes.[3] 100 years ago there was no processed food. Food was cooked from scratch daily. Food was sourced locally and people ate seasonally.

Now, all food can be obtained all year round (often travelling huge distances with the challenges that hold for the planet), and there is a prevalence of processed, packaged and microwaveable foods. This section will explore how to identify real food and the health consequences of an ultra-processed diet.

Over the years, the consumption of meals prepared at home has gradually declined. Convenience is king! The human body is well aware of the difference between homemade dishes and frozen pizza, yet do not take the silence of your body for granted; it reacts and repeatedly communicates in ways you might not immediately notice with symptoms such as bloating, acidity, acid reflux, poor sleep, lack of concentration, low energy levels, constipation, and a number of others when you eat the wrong food.

In recent years, research has shown that adults who frequently consume meals prepared away from home are at higher risk of type 2 diabetes, obesity, heart disease, and premature death.[4] The purpose of this component is to provide practical tips and tools to identify real food and create healthy family habits in your kitchen through the preparation of simple meals.

Component 3C: Create Your Own Meal Plan

It is no secret that diet is the most significant factor affecting your blood glucose levels. Planning your personalised meal plan is one of the best things you can do for your health. By doing this, you will be able to set goals you can reach and be inspired to push further and reach milestones you can be proud of. You are also allowed to fail, bounce back, and try again.

I have laid out this blueprint over four weeks so that it is easier to understand. Each week has three components.

In the first week, you will take a step back and understand where you are by assessing your baseline. This may require some honest introspection as well as some self-reflection in terms of your lifestyle choices.

The second week will help you become familiar with identifying foods based on their nutrients and combining them in the right proportions for your meals.

The third week will teach you how to adjust meals according to your own blood glucose levels.

In the last and fourth week, you will improve the quality of your meal plan and monitor it 24/7 using technology. You will also learn how to prevent setbacks and stay motivated.

Component 4C: Count on Active Movement, Sound Sleep, and Stress Management

A lifestyle change can be defined in many ways; however, when your physician prescribes a lifestyle change, he/she usually refers to changes to dietary habits and physical activity. There is no doubt that the importance of healthy eating and physical activity cannot be overstated. However, the impact of other lifestyle factors, such as sleep and stress management, on blood glucose has also been extensively studied.

Exercise is not something that many people enjoy. Probably because the images of exercise presented in our culture aren't ones that everyone enjoys. For example, gyms, swimming pools, biking, and jogging. In my opinion, exercise is the activity of movement, or as I refer to "active movement" and you have to find something you love to do, something that makes you break out a sweat, and commit to it as you would to a meeting with your dearest friend.

As part of this component, you will learn how to assess your fitness level, set your personal goals, and make fitness a routine part of your life in order to achieve perfect blood glucose levels.

People with type 2 diabetes are four times more likely to suffer from insomnia symptoms than the general population.[5] Poor sleeping habits not only increase the risk of developing type 2 diabetes but also worsen glucose control in a person with diabetes.[6] The 4C suggests techniques and tips for managing sleep disturbances to maintain adequate glucose control.

Stress is a part of everyone's life. Stress management is crucial for having good blood glucose control for people with diabetes, and not just relaxing to feel better.

You will learn how cognitive behavioural therapy can help you to identify and change destructive or disturbing thought patterns that negatively influence your behaviour and emotions. By connecting with family and friends and using positive psychology tips, you will increase your resilience and coping abilities. I will discuss a number of additional ways in which you can manage stress and improve your overall health, as well as adjunct therapies that may be helpful in managing stress.

Component 5C: Capitalise on Technology

A crucial component of your journey toward health and happiness is setting goals and monitoring your progress in order to maintain motivation and remain on track. With today's cutting-edge technology, gadgets, and healthcare solutions, monitoring yourself is easy and convenient. Diabetes is a chronic disease associated with fluctuating blood glucose levels that requires ongoing support and monitoring.

You have to track what you eat and then assess the food's effect on your blood sugar levels. If you take insulin, you have to calculate the correct amount needed to compensate for the number of carbs you've eaten. The 5C introduces you to these technologies (blood glucose meters, continuous glucose monitoring devices, insulin pumps, and smart pens) and teaches you how to use them for your benefit.

Lastly, this journey will give you an opportunity to reconnect with yourself and form a positive relationship with your health and well-being. It might sound hard but once you realise that the power to attain health is in your own hands, it becomes an adventure. The first step is all that matters, as the rest will follow.

Now that you have decided to take care of yourself and your family, sit back, relax, grab a cup of tea or coffee, and let's get started!

Diabetes should not be viewed as a frightening disease but rather as a hurdle you must—and can—overcome to live your life to the fullest!

CHAPTER 2

INSULIN RESISTANCE, PREDIABETES, AND DIABETES

*I*magine a world where you have the power to take control of your health, make informed choices, and live a life free from the limitations imposed by a chronic condition. That world is within your reach, and it begins with understanding diabetes.

Whether you have been diagnosed with diabetes yourself or someone you care about is living with this condition, learning about diabetes is a transformative journey that will empower you to make positive changes and embrace a healthier lifestyle.

Diabetes is more than just a medical term or a set of numbers on a blood test. It's a complex condition that affects millions of people worldwide, impacting their daily lives, relationships, and overall well-being. By investing your time in understanding diabetes, you unlock a world of knowledge and insights that will guide you towards better health outcomes.

Visualise standing at the edge of a wide river, with a desire to cross to the other side. You know that building a bridge is the key to reaching your destination safely. But before you can construct that bridge, you must first gain a deep understanding of the river itself—the flow of its currents, the nature of its obstacles, and the best materials to use for a sturdy and reliable structure.

Now, let's apply this analogy to the journey of managing diabetes and achieving a healthier and happier life. Just as a bridge is essential for traversing a river, knowledge about diabetes is crucial for navigating the complexities of the condition. Understanding what, how, and why diabetes occurs becomes the foundation upon which you can build your bridge towards optimal health.

In simple terms, type 2 diabetes is a chronic disease (long-term) that affects your body's ability to convert food into energy. In order to survive, you need food that provides energy, and the currency of energy is glucose. Nonetheless, glucose requires a hormone called insulin to be able to enter many of the body's cells and release energy.

When the cells are not responding efficiently (resistant) to insulin and hindering the entrance of glucose into the cells, glucose increases in the blood circulation. Over time, you will notice that your blood glucose is higher than normal. This is the manifestation of type 2 diabetes.[7]

Type 2 diabetes begins with insulin resistance in the liver, fat cells and muscle cells. At the beginning of the disease, many diabetics actually have higher insulin levels in the blood than healthy people due to insulin resistance. But as time passes, insulin resistance impairs the body's ability to secrete insulin.

In short, you produce less insulin and your cells resist the little you produce. It results in less glucose in the cells where it is needed and more in the blood, where it is not. It is important to know that type 2 diabetes does not appear overnight. It takes 5-10 years for it to manifest, giving you a window of opportunity for remission with lifestyle changes and weight loss.[8]

Diabetes is not as straightforward as described. There are several dynamic processes that must be understood. I have attempted to make diabetes' what, why, and how as simple as possible.

It's important to understand that "insulin resistance" is the key factor responsible for developing type 2 diabetes. The condition is also the prime culprit in the development of diseases like hypertension, dyslipidemia (high and abnormal levels of fats in the blood, especially bad cholesterol), cardiovascular diseases, and stroke.

Now, you may be wondering what is meant by 'insulin resistance' and 'impaired insulin secretion.' Let's go step by step.

Insulin Resistance
Normal Human Physiology – Diabetes 101

Let's go back to school. Remember when you thought science was boring?! Well, now you're about to prove yourself wrong! A brief look at how glucose and insulin are normally processed or metabolised in your body could help you understand. Your body is a huge chemical laboratory of organic compounds!

Here is a step-by-step look at the chemical changes that occur from the time you eat food until it is burned as fuel. Let's begin with the types of meals we consume and how they are processed.

What Happens When You Eat a Carbohydrate-Rich Meal?

When you eat food that contains carbohydrates for instance, grains, beans, fruits, sugars, and milk (more about these in Chapter 3), the enzymes secreted by your mouth and small intestine (amylase, maltase, lactase, and sucrase) break down long carbohydrate chains (called polysaccharides) to the smallest carbohydrate units (called monosaccharides) like glucose, fructose, and galactose.

These monosaccharides first travel to your liver, where the liver takes them in and converts galactose to glucose, and breaks fructose into even smaller carbon-containing units.

The major portion of food usually consists of carbohydrates that break down to glucose. This glucose—the sugars as you would commonly identify them—can either:

a) be burned as immediate energy,
b) be stored as glycogen in the liver or muscles (for short-term storage), or
c) be converted to fat and stored in adipose tissue (the long-term storage that manifests in our body as 'body fat,' the arch enemy of weight loss).

One of the primary functions of the liver and insulin is to maintain optimal glucose levels in the blood. Not an easy job especially nowadays. This process is quite complex, and tightly controlled by a dynamic hormonal process. In order to make it easier to understand, I will use the analogy of a warehouse operation.

1. To elaborate, let's say that human cells—like those in the liver and muscles—are like smart warehouses. These warehouses store glucose and use it whenever needed to produce energy (ATP). However, these smart warehouses have smart doors that are opened by a smart keycard (insulin). These insulin keycards are produced in the head office (in the islets of Langerhans cells inside the pancreas) and released based on the load of glucose received.

   Whenever we eat carbohydrate-rich foods, glucose molecules are broken down, which move towards the warehouse (cells) for storage as glycogen or used as energy. The larger the carbohydrate meal, the higher the volume of smartcards (insulin) required to open the smart doors.

   But every warehouse has a certain capacity, and what happens when the load is beyond the storage capacity of the warehouse? If the warehouses are jam-packed with glucose molecules or unable to take in glucose molecules as they refuse the smartcards, the glucose-loaded trucks outside wait for the door to open.

   But since the insulin key cards don't seem to be working as they are controlled by a feedback mechanism, the trucks ask the head office—the pancreas—for assistance, but all they get in return is more insulin key cards.

   Do you see the issue now? Resistance to insulin leads to increased insulin concentration, called an "insulin resistant" state. Lack of insulin means that the muscles 'starve' because the glucose does not enter the cells at the right rate. There is not as much glucose inside the muscles as there should be. Eventually, we end up with loads of glucose and insulin in the blood this gradual increase in the concentration of glucose in the blood over time is diabetes.

2. Now, let us understand why the warehouses refuse access to insulin keycards. The causes of this resistance are many: weight gain, types of foods, lack of physical movement, stress, hormonal changes, and sleeping habits, to name a few. (We will discuss them in the upcoming chapters.)

3. The human body is so well-prepared to fire-fight that it has its contingency plan ready. When the liver and muscle cells cannot use the excess glucose in the blood, the trucks move to the additional storage, the adipose tissue. These adipose tissue 'warehouses' are also operated with these insulin key cards, hence they take in glucose, convert it into fat molecules, and store them.

However, this process is not as simple as described above, as having either too much or too little glucose in the blood can have serious health consequences.

Figure 2.1: Illustration of insulin resistance causing blood glucose spike

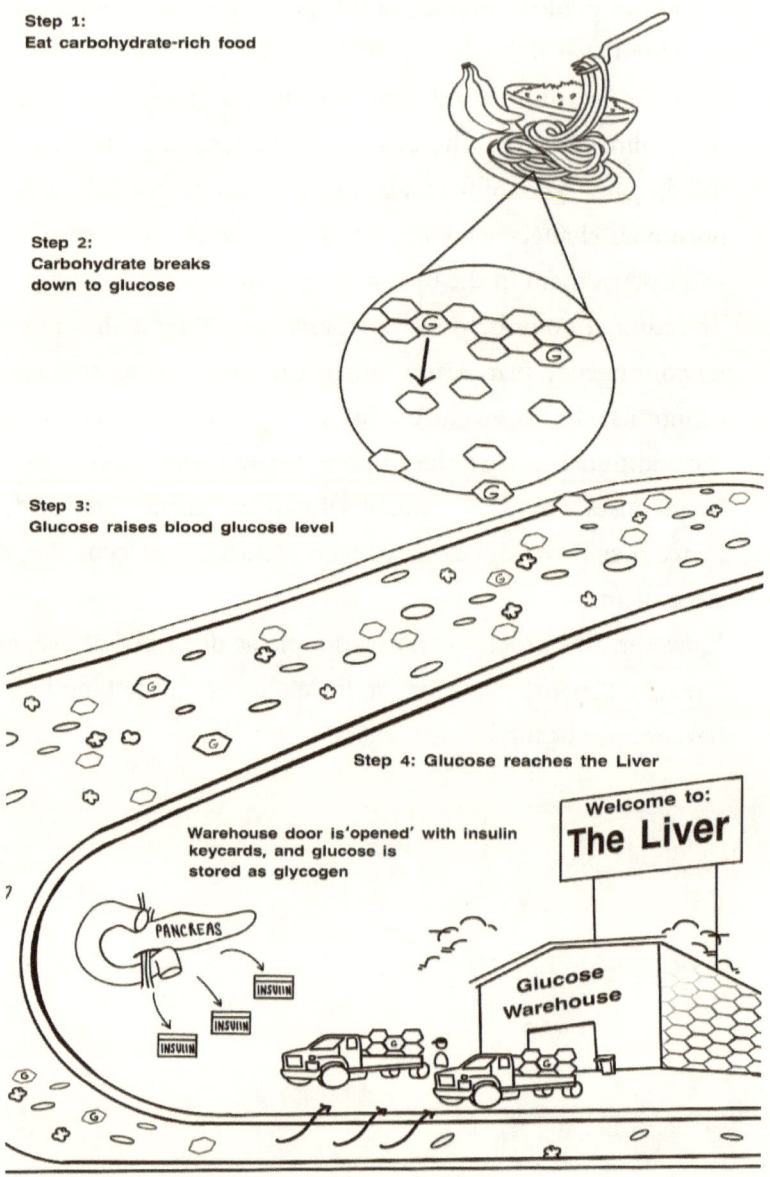

Insulin Resistance, Prediabetes, and Diabetes

Step 5:
Now what if the warehouse is <u>full</u>

Step 6:
Insulin secretion increases while glucose accumulates

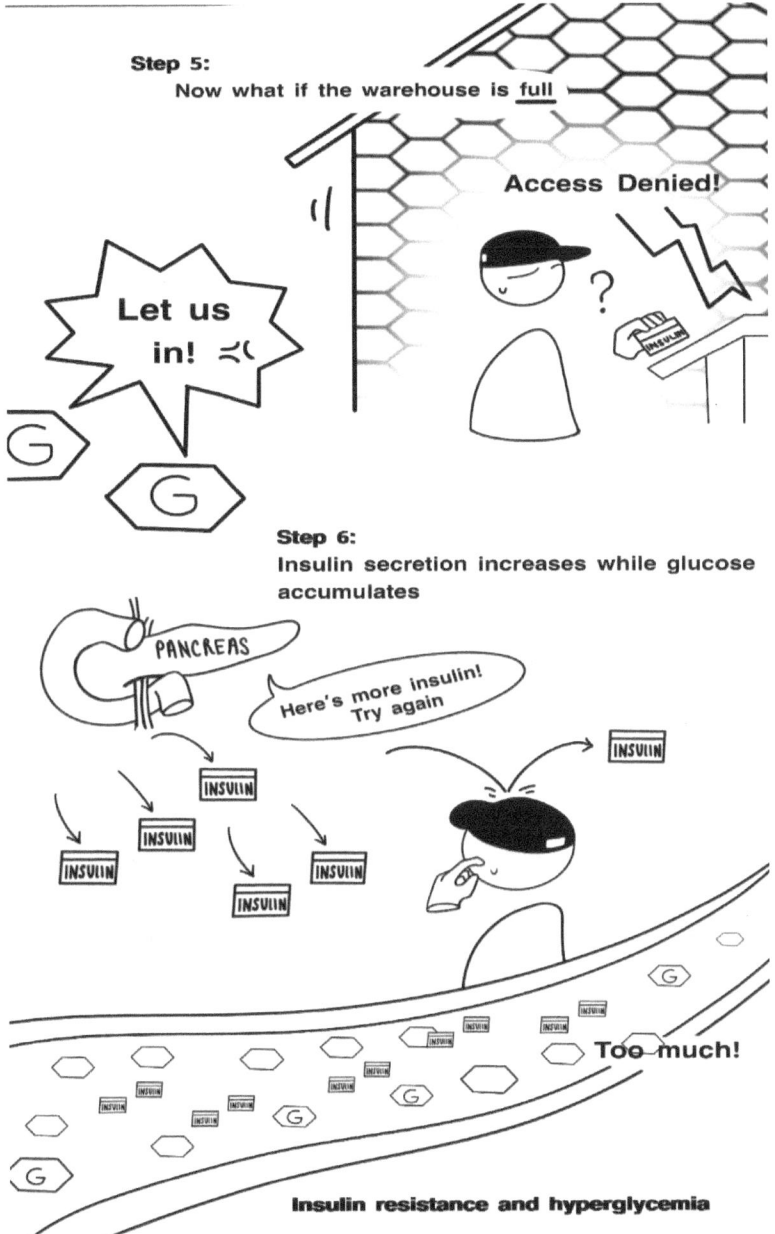

Insulin resistance and hyperglycemia

Insulin - How Does it Work?

Your pancreas contains highly specialised cells called beta cells (β-cells). These beta cells are found in the clusters called the "islets of Langerhans" and are the only cells in your body capable of producing insulin. Insulin acts as a key to opening millions of cellular doors found on the surface of the cells for the entry of glucose. So, insulin is a vital hormone for the normal functioning of our body. When the glucose levels rise in the blood, the beta cells release insulin in a biphasic manner (in two phases).

The first phase consists of a brief spike lasting about ten minutes to help your liver uptake glucose from the blood. This cycle is followed by the second phase, in which the insulin release for absorption of larger amounts of glucose in circulation reaches a plateau or a steady glucose level for around 2–3 hours. It means that insulin levels increase after eating a carbohydrate-rich meal and remain in the blood circulation for two to three hours following the meal to assist in the absorption of glucose by cells.[9]

Now, the glucose released by the food is first absorbed by the liver and muscle cells to be used immediately as a source of energy in tiny "furnaces" called mitochondria. If the cells do not need energy at the time, the excess amounts of glucose are converted to glycogen (a complex chain of glucose molecules). In this stage after your meal, there is approximately 100g of glycogen in the liver and 400g of glycogen in your muscles.

Further, if excessive glucose remains in the blood, it gets converted to fatty acids (tiny droplets of fat). It is stored in the adipose tissue with the help of the same hormone. Insulin now functions as the fat-storage hormone, although fatty acids can also enter the tissues without insulin.

What Happens When You Eat a Fatty Meal?

When your meal contains oil or fat, it travels down to the stomach and duodenum to be broken down into smaller units (called fatty acids) and enters the small intestine for absorption. Ninety percent of this broken-down food is absorbed via the lymphatic system.

The lymphatic system is the supplementary branch of your blood circulation system that consists of blood serum, aids in immunity, and carries a lot of nutrients to most of the body cells from the blood. Once your lymph or blood serum absorbs fats, they rapidly appear in your blood. Now, you understand why your doctor wants to test your cholesterol levels, too, if you have diabetes.

When the fat reaches your liver and muscle cells, it is absorbed into the cells with or without insulin. Once they are inside the cells, they are either burned for energy or stored as fuel for later use in the form of lipid droplets (free fatty acids).

The catch here is that the human body is designed to survive extreme conditions and adapt to starvation. Hence, your cells continue to take in the fatty acids from the circulation until there is no more in the blood. Consequently, your cells are loaded with fat droplets as stored energy if you have a fatty meal.

If you consistently take in more glucose and fatty acids than can be used, it is stored in the 'fat cells' (adipose tissue). However, increasing adipose tissue increases inflammation (when your body activates your immune system by sending out inflammatory cells). This, in turn, triggers the risk of insulin resistance, type 2 diabetes, obesity, cardiovascular disease, hypertension, and certain cancers.

Moreover, in a situation where the 'normal' fat mass storage capacity is full, the fat settles in places where it shouldn't be. So-called ectopic fat. For example, in the pancreas where it affects insulin production, and in the liver where it causes fatty liver etc.

Although the consumption of fat does not in itself lead to increased insulin secretion, saturated fats have been shown to increase insulin resistance. According to an interesting study published in Diabetes Care in 2020, 16 overweight men consumed a saturated fat-rich diet for four weeks. They ended up with increased liver fat content and increased blood glucose and insulin levels after the meal.

However, when the same men were given a diet with high sugar content, the glucose spike was not as significant.[10] This might suggest that a diet high in saturated fat is more detrimental to metabolic health than a diet high in free sugar, although neither a great for health. Research studies have shown that insulin receptors become less functional within hours of a single high-fat meal, causing glucose to pile in the blood circulation.[1]

It appears that insulin resistance starts in the hypothalamus causing a disruption in the balance of satiety and hunger signals.[12] Of course, this leads to overconsumption of calories; if you don't feel full, you keep eating. Although excess calories can be theoretically stored safely in the adipose tissue, as inflammation increases in this organ and insulin resistance develops in the fat cells, the ability to safely store excess fat is compromised.

One of the consequences of insulin resistance in the adipose tissue is that excess fat is released into the bloodstream and is sequestered by other organs (liver and skeletal muscles) that are not equipped to safely store this excess fat.

This is the start of lipotoxicity. With increased lipotoxicity, the metabolism and energy generation becomes compromised, and the development of chronic diseases (type 2 diabetes, heart disease, and polycystic ovary syndrome) associated with insulin resistance becomes accelerated. The levels of fat in the diet and the composition of those fatty acids in the mix can have a significant role in the modulation of insulin resistance.

How Does Your Body Respond to a Meal High in Fat and Carbohydrate?

When you consume a meal that is high in fat and simple carbohydrates (for example, pizza, burger, cookies, French fries, or donuts), the fat content appears before the glucose in the blood during the digestion process. Your liver and muscles absorb them because they cannot refuse them.

Let's go back to the warehouse analogy. A warehouse that is full of stock will refuse to accept any more supplies. Hence, your body cells send signals to block the gates by not giving access to insulin once it is full of glucose intake. The fat got in through the back door; nobody saw it because it didn't need the insulin key.

Eventually, what remains outside the warehouse (cells) are piles of immediate energy sources, that is, the excess glucose and the invalid insulin keycards or *insulin*. Although your muscles and liver are designed to store a large amount of glycogen and a small amount of fat, they end up rejecting insulin after a heavy fatty-starchy meal. This rejection is called insulin resistance. High blood glucose (hyperglycemia) and high blood insulin (hyperinsulinemia) are the conditions that follow.

It is not the insulin per se but the excessive accumulation of insulin and consequential high glucose concentrations caused by insulin resistance that triggers severe metabolic dysfunction and increases your risk of chronic diseases like type 2 diabetes, fatty liver, and heart diseases.

What Happens After the Fat Enters Your Adipose Tissue?

Another reason for insulin resistance is increased body fat, body weight, and obesity. The adipose tissue is located in many places in the human body, for instance, the abdomen, thighs, buttocks, face, and chest, to name a few. These tissues are designed to absorb the excessive fat content with the help of the enzyme lipase. The fatty acid transports proteins and stores them for a long period; this is not a dead warehouse of fat cells. The fat cells protect your organs. However, excessive fat storage in these adipose tissue cells causes low-grade inflammation—a constantly stressful situation. The situation also triggers another set of reactions that further increase insulin resistance.

Other Reasons for Insulin Resistance

Genetic predisposition also plays a vital role. Some people inherit a set of genes from their parents that make their tissues resistant to insulin. However, genetic predisposition only loads the gun! This means that even though you have a family history of type 2 diabetes, the occurrence of type 2 diabetes can be delayed and even avoided if you make optimum lifestyle choices. In conclusion, insulin resistance is triggered by lifestyle factors like a diet high in simple carbohydrates, a high-fat diet, increasing body weight, physical inactivity, and chronic stress.

Beta-Cell Dysfunction

Insulin resistance is assumed to be a major feature of type 2 diabetes. However, the other crucial factor that leads to it, is impaired insulin secretion due to the poor function of the beta-cells in the pancreas that produce insulin. You know now that insulin must be produced from the beta-cells in order for the glucose to be allowed into the cells. But these beta cells are highly sensitive to the accumulation of excessive fat in them. The collection of excess fat in your beta cells causes severe dysfunction, known as lipotoxicity or fat poisoning.

On the one hand, the beta cells are tired of producing excessive insulin, and on the other hand, they are abused by excessive fat accumulation. Consequently, the death of beta-cells (apoptosis) exhausts the body's capacity to produce sufficient, or indeed any, insulin, resulting in type 2 diabetes. However, the time taken for this process may vary from months to years depending on several other factors in the body and it varies from person to person.

It is important to note that your body stops producing new beta cells after the age of twenty, and consequently, you have a limited reserve of beta cells for life. Extensive research has revealed that more than half of the beta-cell population die when type 2 diabetes is clinically diagnosed (i.e. when your doctor says you have diabetes).[13]

Therefore, it is vital that you use wisely and efficiently the remaining functional beta cells. Not only must you adopt healthy lifestyle choices that will reduce insulin resistance, but you must also limit triggers that cause a spike in blood sugar, triggering a rush of insulin (such as a diet high in saturated fat and simple sugars).

Diabetes – What Happens With Obesity?

Having too much body fat can lead to type 2 diabetes, and the risk of developing this disease rises as your body mass index (BMI) increases. As obesity becomes more common worldwide, the number of people with type 2 diabetes has also risen.

The connection between obesity and type 2 diabetes is complex and involves various changes in the body. These changes affect beta cells' function, how adipose tissue (fat tissue) behaves, and the body's ability to use insulin effectively.

Hence, the International Diabetes Federation (IDF) has recommended that people diagnosed with prediabetes should be encouraged to focus on lifestyle modifications to achieve at least a 5% to 7% weight reduction and increased physical activity to prevent type 2 diabetes[14] from developing. A 5% weight loss reduces the risk of developing type 2 diabetes by 50% and a

10% weight loss reduces the risk by 80%.[15] Did you know that shedding just one kilogram of weight can have a remarkable impact on reducing the risk of type 2 diabetes? According to a study published in Diabetes Care, even a modest weight loss of one kilogram can lead to a significant 16% decrease in the risk of developing type 2 diabetes. This finding highlights the power of small changes in your health journey.[16]

As you adopt the 5C lifestyle prescription, you will develop your own plan to reduce insulin resistance. As a result of the changes you will make, excessive fat accumulation will be prevented in tissues that are not designed to store fat, and glucose and insulin spikes will be prevented in the blood, meaning the beta cells will not be damaged further.

Types of Diabetes

There are several types of diabetes which cause your blood glucose equilibrium to be diminished. You will read about different types of diabetes throughout this book. Let's clarify the differences between each type of diabetes.

Prediabetes

Prediabetes is not a type of diabetes itself, but rather a warning sign or a precursor to type 2 diabetes. Type 2 diabetes is not an acute disease that suddenly appears, lasts for a short time, and goes away. It is a chronic disease manifested due to low-grade abuse of your body for 5-10 years or more. Prediabetes refers to a condition where blood glucose levels are higher than normal, but not high enough to be diagnosed as type 2 diabetes.

It is an early warning sign on your journey toward developing diabetes and potential complications. This condition is often underplayed by medical professionals who are focused on treating existing diseases.

Indeed, when my friend mentioned her prediabetes diagnosis to a nurse, the nurse replied, "Whatever that is! I have never heard of prediabetes." Shocking, isn't it? Although there is no medication for 'prediabetes' but the importance of lifestyle intervention in reversing this condition is clearly not emphasised enough.

This condition occurs when your liver and muscle cells are becoming resistant to insulin's signals to allow glucose into them, causing a bottleneck situation in glucose absorption. Hence, the levels of glucose in the blood remain marginally elevated. You may be considered prediabetic if your fasting blood glucose falls between 100-125 mg/dl (5.6-6.9 mmol/L) or if your haemoglobin A1C is between 6.0-6.4% (39-47 mmol/mol).

However, the good news is that we have extensive evidence that changing lifestyle choices and weight loss can prevent the growth of prediabetes into full-blown type 2 diabetes.

Figure 2.2: Natural History of type 2 diabetes (Adapted from Holman RR, 1999) [17]

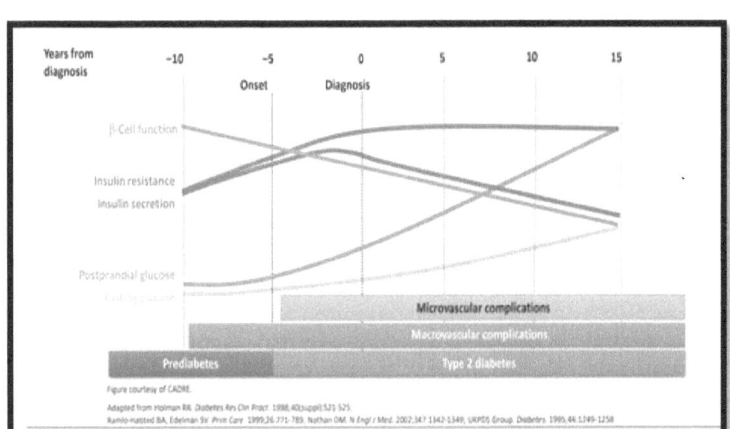

Type 2 Diabetes

Type 2 diabetes, previously referred to as 'non-insulin-dependent diabetes' or 'adult-onset diabetes,' accounts for 90–95% of all diabetes in the world. It occurs when your pancreatic beta cells lose the ability to produce sufficient insulin while your liver and muscles become insulin resistant (lethargic) to glucose absorption. It is a double whammy where there is little insulin for glucose absorption, and when glucose reaches the cells for absorption, the doors resist opening. This leads to high blood glucose and the consequences of this excessive glucose on heart, eye, kidney and nerve health.

Hence, the day you know you have type 2 diabetes, much of the damage has already occurred, but taking medications to control hyperglycemia may delay complications.

However, until and unless you reach the root cause of the problem to treat insulin resistance, symptomatic treatment is incomplete. In the last decade, robust research studies have shown that lifestyle changes can slow the progression of your diabetes, reverse its effect by a few years, and even eliminate the condition in some cases.

At least initially, and often throughout their lifetime, these individuals may not need insulin therapy or support to survive. However, when beta cells have overproduced insulin for an extended period and no longer function properly, managing blood glucose is accomplished with exogenous insulin (insulin that comes from outside through injections or other means) and oral medications.

Suppose you are diagnosed with type 2 diabetes with insulin resistance, lifestyle modifications with diet and increased physical activity are proven to be your ticket to maintaining good glycemic control and becoming non-diabetic in some cases.

Gestational Diabetes

Gestational diabetes mellitus (GDM) is a common pregnancy complication in which spontaneous high blood glucose develops. It is diagnosed in the second or third trimester of pregnancy (ranging between 24 to 28 weeks of pregnancy) and was not overt before pregnancy. This diabetes poses a severe threat to maternal and child health.

Much like prediabetes, gestational diabetes is often a sign of the undiagnosed or unmanifested dysfunction of the beta cells and insulin resistance, in simple words, an alarm of future type 2 diabetes. The damage, malfunction, and death of the beta cells and the effects of insulin resistance become evident only as the pregnancy hormones add to the conditions of insulin resistance.[18]

The International Diabetes Federation (IDF) reports that half of the women who have had GDM could develop type 2 diabetes within five to ten years after delivery which increases the risk of obesity and type 2 diabetes in the unborn child too.[19] One of my research studies, published in the British Medical Journal in 2022, evidently shows that a 12-week of moderate-intensity lifestyle intervention in early pregnancy could reduce the risk of GDM by 41 % in high-risk pregnant women.[20]

I have shared with you these lifestyle changes in the 5C program. These changes reduce excessive weight gain during pregnancy by reducing cravings for unhealthy foods, improving motivation to exercise, and improving overall well-being.

Type 1 Diabetes

Type 1 diabetes, which was previously known as 'insulin-dependent diabetes' or 'juvenile-onset diabetes,' has traditionally affected children and teenagers and accounts for 5-10% of diabetes. It is a serious condition where your blood glucose level is too high because your body can't make insulin. This happens because your body attacks its own beta cells in the pancreas (autoimmune disease).

When you have type 1 diabetes, your body still breaks down the carbohydrates from food and drinks and turns them into glucose. But when the glucose enters your bloodstream, there's no insulin to allow it into your body's cells. More and more glucose then builds up in your bloodstream, leading to high blood sugar levels.

As a result, exogenous insulin (insulin injected through a syringe, pen, or insulin pump) is needed to maintain healthy blood glucose levels.

Less Common Types of Diabetes

1. Monogenic Diabetes Syndromes

These are rare and usually inherited forms of diabetes, caused by a faulty gene, accounting for up to 4% of all cases. Examples are Neonatal Diabetes and Maturity-Onset Diabetes of the Young (MODY).[21] The gene can be inherited from one or both parents or occasionally develop on its own.

2. Cystic Fibrosis and Pancreatitis-Related Diabetes

Cystic fibrosis is an inherited genetic disorder in which the lungs and the digestive system get clogged with mucus. Pancreatitis is a condition in which the pancreas becomes inflamed, which can be very painful in the short term and could lead to complications including secondary diabetes. Alcohol abuse and gall stones are the main risk factors for pancreatitis.

3. Drug or Chemical-Induced Diabetes

This type of diabetes is developed with the use of, or emergency administration of, such anti-infective drugs, cardiovascular drugs, and hormonal drugs.

Recognising The Early Signs of Diabetes

As discussed earlier, type 2 diabetes is a chronic progressive disease and does not give clear symptoms until high blood sugar levels are reached. The early symptoms of diabetes could be evident for some; however, they may remain unnoticed by others.

The symptoms of type 2 diabetes tend to come on more gradually than type 1 diabetes. There may be no symptoms in the early stages of diabetes. Type 1 and type 2 diabetes have some symptoms that are the same and some that are different.

Early Warning Symptoms

The American Diabetes Association recommends seeing your doctor for blood sugar tests if you have any of the following general warning signs of diabetes:

- Extreme thirst (polydipsia)
- Frequent urination, especially at night (polyuria)
- Unintentional weight loss
- Increased hunger (polyphagia)
- Blurred vision
- Numbness or tingling in your hands and feet
- Fatigue
- Skin that's very itchy or dry
- Wounds that don't heal quickly

The above symptoms can easily be missed or attributed to other causes—for example, menopause, Fibromyalgia or other immune disorders, or even depression. Often in type 2 diabetes, these symptoms are mild and might take several years to be noticed.

Any of these symptoms which persist for more than a couple of weeks should not be ignored, and a doctor's appointment should be sought.

Other Warning Signs of Type 1 Diabetes

Type 1 diabetes symptoms can develop quickly, even within a few weeks or months. In addition to the symptoms outlined above, you may experience additional symptoms such as:

- Sudden, unintentional weight loss
- Wetting the bed after a history of being dry at night
- Yeast infection in a prepubescent girl
- Breath that smells like fruit
- Flu-like symptoms, including nausea, vomiting, problems breathing, and loss of consciousness (diabetic ketoacidosis- this condition is a medical emergency and requires immediate medical treatment)

Are you at risk of diabetes?

You can take a 60-second online test to know your risk of type 2 diabetes and prediabetes on the following links:

(https://www.diabetes.org/risk-test)

https://riskscore.diabetes.org.uk/start

https://www.cdc.gov/prediabetes/pdf/Prediabetes-Risk-Test-Final.pdf

Also, find below the list of risk factors for diabetes, although the list is not exhaustive.

Type of Diabetes	*Who is at risk*
Type 1	- Children - Young adults - Those with an immediate relative with type 1 diabetes
Type 2	- Being over age 45 - Being overweight or obese - Having a sedentary lifestyle - Being a smoker - Having a family history of diabetes - Having high blood pressure - Having a low level of HDL 'good' cholesterol, or a high level of triglycerides - Being of certain ethnic backgrounds, such as American Indian, American Asian, Alaskan Native, Hispanic, or Black - Having a history of gestational diabetes or a recent delivery of a baby weighing 9 pounds/4kg or more - Having polycystic ovary syndrome (PCOS) - Having acanthosis nigricans—dark, thick, and velvety skin around your neck or armpits

How does the physician conclude that you have diabetes?

Your doctor will ask you questions about your symptoms and likely run some blood tests.

Several tests can diagnose diabetes. These include:

- **HbA1C (Glycated haemoglobin):** This test shows your blood glucose level has averaged for the last 2 or 3 months; this does not require you to fast or drink anything.
- **Fasting Plasma Glucose (FPG):** You will need to fast (no calorie intake) for at least 8 hours before this test is done, and at least 2 elevated values are needed to make the diagnosis
- **Oral Glucose Tolerance test (OGTT):** This test takes 2 to 3 hours. Your blood glucose levels are tested initially and then repeated at intervals for 2 hours after you've consumed a specific sweet drink. The 2-hour postprandial glucose test should be performed using a glucose load containing 75-g anhydrous glucose dissolved in water.
- **Random Plasma Glucose Test:** You can have this test done at any time and do not need to be fasting.

Insulin Resistance, Prediabetes, and Diabetes

The table below outlines most guidelines that use the standard diagnostic criteria proposed by American Diabetes Association (ADA).[22]

Table 2.2 Diagnostic criteria for diabetes

Test	Normal	Prediabetes	Diabetes
Fasting glucose	Less than 100 mg/dL	100-125 mg/dL	≥ 126 mg/dL
	Less than 5.6 mmol/L	5.6 – 6.9 mmol/L	≥ 7.0 mmol/L
OR 2-hour glucose following ingestion of 75-g oral glucose load	Less than 140 mg/dL	140-199 mg/dL	≥200 mg/dL
	< 7.8 mmol/L	≥ 7.8 and 11.1 mmol/L	≥ 11.1 mmol/L
OR random plasma glucose in a symptomatic patient	Less than 140 mg/dL	NA	≥200 mg/dL
	< 7.8 mmol/L	NA	≥ 11.1 mmol/L
OR HbA1c	Less than 5.7%	5.7 – 6.4%	≥6.5%
	Less than 39 mmol/mol	39 - 47 mmol/mol	≥ 48 mmol/mol

The easiest way to convert blood glucose from mg/dL to mmol/L is to divide the value in mg/dL with conversion factor 18 and change the units. However, glycated haemoglobin (HbA1c) is considered a diagnostic test, particularly in those who are very likely to have the disease.

Diabetes can be reversed: But conditions apply

In a nutshell, type 2 diabetes starts with excessive fat accumulation in tissues not designed to store excessive ectopic fat, inducing insulin resistance, followed by increased insulin secretion. At the same time, it destroys the insulin-producing beta cells causing a gradual increase in fasting blood glucose and post-meal blood glucose. Eventually, this issue develops into hyperglycemia (high blood glucose)—full-blown type 2 diabetes.

To treat insulin resistance you must address the root cause of the problem. Weight gain is one of the strongest causes of insulin resistance. In the last decade, robust research studies have shown that significant weight loss can reverse its effect for a few years and may even eliminate insulin resistance in some cases.

As such, calling it "diabetes reversal" would be unfair since it implies that it is permanent, although no guarantee exists that it will last. We do not have enough research to say that this is a permanent solution to type 2 diabetes, but you may be able to put it into "remission." This means your blood sugar levels are below the diabetes range, so you are not required to take diabetes medicine. And this could be life-changing.

According to the International Experts on Diabetes in 2021, people with type 2 diabetes should be considered in remission after sustaining normal blood glucose (sugar) levels for three months or more-although the duration is not definitively established yet.

Which is when your HbA1c—a measure of long-term blood glucose levels—remains below 6.5% (48mmol/mol) for at least three months, without diabetes medication.[23]

Diabetes remission may be achieved through lifestyle changes, medical or surgical interventions, or a combination of these approaches.

What are the conditions required to put diabetes into remission?

1. People with type 1 diabetes cannot put their diabetes into remission. Even so, scientists are working hard to discover how this might be possible and to develop new treatments.
2. Remission in type 2 Diabetes is achievable for those who are overweight or obese and who lose a substantial amount of weight (around 15kg or 5-15% of body weight) safely, as research has shown this is most effective. However, ongoing research is actively working toward finding out if remission from type 2 diabetes is possible for people with lower body weight.
3. Early diagnosis and intervention are crucial for successful remission of type 2 diabetes. These interventions are most effective when executed during a 6-year therapeutic window when the pancreatic β-cells (cells that release insulin) remain functional.[24]
4. Rapid weight loss is not advised if you are under 18, pregnant, breastfeeding or have ever been diagnosed with an eating disorder. Considering remission during these phases could not be a safe option.

5. Achieving remission requires motivation and commitment to lifestyle changes. In the past few years, there have been strong research studies indicating that intensive low-calorie meal plans of around 850 calories with meal replacement drinks have the potential to achieve this goal.
6. A gradual approach to weight loss has also shown promising results. Weight loss through a Mediterranean diet or a low-carbohydrate diet is also reported to bring about remission.[26]
7. Interestingly, oral medications of GLP1 and GLP1/GIP agonists used in diabetes, and also used alone in obesity and prediabetes have recently been shown to provide dramatic weight loss that dramatically reduces the risk of developing diabetes.[26, 27]
8. Alternatively, weight loss through bariatric surgery procedures of Roux-en-Y gastric bypass (RYGB), sleeve gastrectomy (SG), and One Anastomosis Gastric Bypass can result in significant weight loss and remission in the early years.[28]
9. Those with poor glucose control, increased diabetes complications, advanced age and low C-peptide levels (indicating decreased endogenous insulin production) have not shown effective remission in the trials.

Don't forget! That remission is not a one-off, once-and-for-all event. It needs to be maintained because there's always a chance that your diabetes might return. Keeping an eye on your weight, and adjusting your eating pattern and activity level if it creeps up again, is key to long-term success.

Even if it doesn't put you into remission, losing weight and making the right dietary choices, moving more, sleeping well, and relaxing will certainly help to slow down any movement towards heart, eye, nerve, and kidney complications.

Remember, it's your life and your lifestyle choices are yours to make.

Diabetes medications: how do they work?

When lifestyle modifications, dietary regimes, behavioural and self-management therapies, and exercise routines are not sufficient to control the symptoms of a newly diagnosed person with diabetes, oral medication is added to control the blood glucose levels.

If you are already on medication, then the right lifestyle choices will help you keep your list of medications shorter and prevent complications. Diabetes medications work in several different ways. These medications improve the effectiveness of the body's natural insulin sensitivity (reduce insulin resistance), limit blood sugar production from the liver, increase insulin production, and enhance blood glucose absorption.

If you are prescribed medications for diabetes, it is important that you understand how they work on your body. Always take your medicine exactly as your doctor prescribes it. Discuss your specific questions and concerns with your healthcare provider only. When taking your medication, be mindful of what and when you are taking it. Listed in the appendix are the most common medications recommended by the American Diabetes Association, but it's best to discuss your medication options with your treating physician.[29] (Appendix III)

Take Home Message

- Type 2 diabetes is not an acute disease that suddenly appears, lasts for a short time, and goes away. It is a chronic disease manifested due to low-grade abuse of your body for 5-10 years or more.
- There is no doubt that genetics makes you susceptible to type 2 diabetes, but lifestyle choices play a crucial role in triggering your vulnerability. It is genetics that load the gun, but it is lifestyle choices that trigger or hold the trigger.
- Type 2 diabetes starts with excessive fat accumulation in tissues not designed to store excessive ectopic fat, inducing insulin resistance, followed by increased insulin secretion. At the same time, it destroys the insulin-producing beta cells causing a gradual increase in fasting blood glucose and post-meal blood glucose. Eventually, this issue develops into hyperglycemia (high blood glucose) and full-blown type 2 diabetes.
- Diabetes remission may be achieved through lifestyle changes, medical or surgical interventions, or a combination of these approaches.

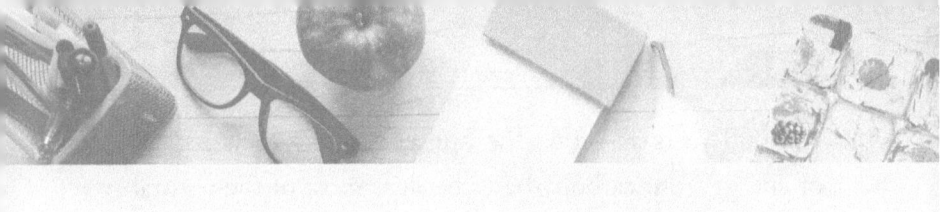

CHAPTER 3

CARBS AND FAT METABOLISM—AND WHY THEY MATTER!

Dietary Carbohydrates 101

Have you ever wondered why you love carbohydrates, whether it's the comforting taste of bread, the satisfying feeling of rice, or the irresistible allure of sweets? Giving up carbohydrates can be an uphill battle. But why?

The truth is there's a complex interplay between the human body and carbohydrates that makes them incredibly difficult to resist. At the core of it all lies the fact that our bodies are inherently wired to run on carbohydrates as their primary source of fuel. While protein and fat can also be used for energy, carbohydrates are like the smoothest, most seamless, and "smoke-free" fuel option for our extraordinary biological engines.

Your pet dog or cat likes the taste of protein in meat, but humans are primarily drawn to the taste of carbohydrates-sweetness. It is reported that early man was attracted to this natural force around

100,000 years ago too. The hunter-gatherer diets had 30-35% of energy from carbohydrates because most of the natural sweet things are non-poisonous and provide instant energy.[30]

Children and adults both rely heavily on carbohydrates for their energy requirements. Our health begins with carbohydrates at birth when approximately 40% of the energy supplied by milk is carbohydrates (lactose), the most abundant source of energy in the body. Meanwhile, data provided by the Food and Agriculture Organization (FAO) indicates that adults consume about 40-80 percent of their calories as carbohydrates from grains, beans, fruits, vegetables, and milk across different countries.[31]

Essentially, diabetes is a metabolic disorder caused by impaired carbohydrate metabolism or, to be more precise, glucose metabolism. Dietary carbohydrates are composed largely of glucose molecules, which control blood glucose levels. Diabetes management and carbohydrate alteration have been strongly associated since diabetes was first discovered.

In 1797, Dr. John Rollo successfully treated a person with diabetes by prescribing a diet of moderation, consisting primarily of meat and fat. Over the centuries, physiologic experimentation and clinical experience have evolved the carbohydrate-restricted diet in different ways.

During the 1940s, diets high in carbohydrates gained popularity due to increased energy levels, decreased hunger, and improved compliance. During the early 2000s, when the Atkins diet was first becoming more popular, carbohydrates were widely recognized as a trigger for diseases such as diabetes, heart disease, obesity, and cancer. It was followed by an influx of literature proposing that carbohydrates are to blame for diabetes and that eliminating carbohydrates is one simple way to cure the disease.

Nevertheless, the American Dietetic Association guidelines (ADA) stated in 2014 that carbohydrates are important sources of energy, fibre, vitamins, and minerals and should be consumed from vegetables, fruits, whole grains, legumes, and dairy products rather than sugar.[32]

However, monitoring the quantity and quality of carbohydrate intake remains a key strategy in achieving glycaemic control. Moreover, the diet should be individualised based on individual needs, existing eating patterns, preferences, and metabolic goals. In 2020, the ADA reaffirmed these statements.[33]

In spite of this, there is a fear of carbohydrates within the diabetes community. Diets such as low-carb, keto, and no-carb are often discussed, and supermarket shelves are stocked with products with no sugar, low sugar, low carb, and low Glycemic index (GI).

It is essential to understand how dietary carbohydrates are broken down and how they affect blood glucose levels before making an informed decision about carbohydrates. Your questions about sugar, refined carbohydrates, complex carbohydrates, the glycemic index, and dietary fibre will be clarified once you grasp the concept of dietary carbohydrates.

Dietary Carbohydrates

Carbohydrates are probably the most abundant and widespread organic substances in nature, so how do they come into existence? When green plants photosynthesise, carbohydrates are created from carbon dioxide and water, and they are used as a source of energy in leaves, roots, fruits, seeds, stalks, and even the pith under the trunk.

Consequently, we see that most plant-based food sources are high in carbohydrates, such as grains, fruits, vegetables, beans, and nuts. Aside from plants, milk and yoghurt also contain carbohydrates as milk sugars (lactose/milk sugars).

Imagine carbohydrate structure as a string composed of just three types of beads: glucose (G), galactose (Gl), and fructose (F). However, it's important to note that glucose (G) is the most prevalent bead in the string. With this understanding, you have the freedom to string these beads together in countless permutations and combinations. You could create a molecule with G-Gl, G-F, G-G-F, F-F, or even construct a lengthy word-like sequence, such as G-G-G-G-G-G. The possibilities are as vast as your imagination allows.

Using the same analogy, a single bead is a monosaccharide, a string of two beads is a disaccharide, and more than two beads constitute a polysaccharide carbohydrate. In common usage, sugar refers to monosaccharides and disaccharides.

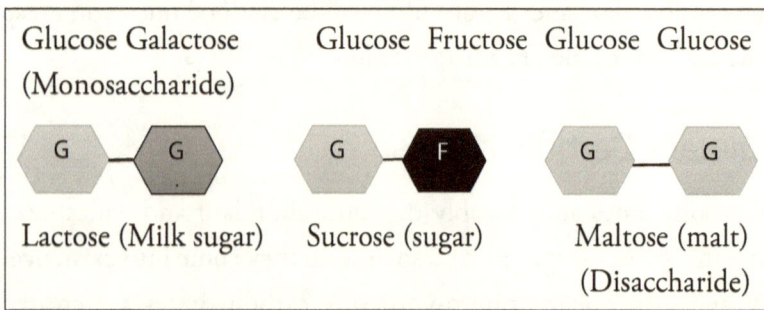

As we discussed, carbohydrates are nothing more than chains of monosaccharide molecules. Mostly the term "sugar" is synonymously used for mono and disaccharides for easy terminology. For example, when we say fruit sugar, we refer to (F + G), milk sugar (lactose G + Gl), and table sugar (sucrose G+ F).

Going back to carbohydrates that are produced in plants and stored in different forms, they exist as a whole food in a complex three-dimensional matrix of many other nutrients, phytochemicals (biologically active compounds found in plants), and fibre. Your digestive system has the ability to interpret, unpackage, absorb and distribute to the tissues in your body.

In short, carbohydrates are essential nutrients that are responsible for the production of energy in the body. They form part of the three main macronutrients, other than proteins and fats. However, there is always some confusion with the terms attached to categorising carbohydrates. For instance, simple and complex carbohydrates, refined and unrefined carbohydrates, or whole carbohydrates.

Let's clear the clutter to understand the real meaning of these words and avoid confusion when choosing carbohydrates.

Simple Carbohydrate vs. Complex Carbohydrate

Primarily carbohydrates were commonly divided into either "simple" or "complex." Simple carbohydrates are made of one or two beads (monosaccharide, disaccharide). These are easily and quickly used for energy by the body because of their simple chemical structure, often leading to a faster rise in blood sugar and insulin secretion from the pancreas which can have negative health effects.

For example, fruits and vegetables consist of simple carbohydrates like glucose and fructose. However, they are encapsulated in a matrix structure that is rich in dietary fibre, vitamins and minerals, and phytonutrients. Another example is milk. Milk and milk products contain lactose, which is a type of simple carbohydrate. These foods do not contain fibre but are rich in protein, calcium, and vitamin D.

Figure 3.2: Simplified scheme summarising the role of the food matrix in digestion and absorption

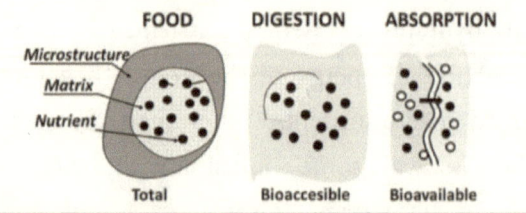

(Source: Aguilera JM, 2019)

Simple carbohydrates that have a negative effect on your health are processed foods with the addition of sucrose, fructose corn syrup, molasses, and dextrose. These elements added to natural foods like fruits, vegetables or grains, create fruit juices, sugary cereals, granola, sodas, sauces, crackers, and bread.

Alternatively, food items with complex carbohydrates have more complex chemical structures, with three or more monosaccharides linked together (known as oligosaccharides and polysaccharides) (Table 3.1). Many complex carbohydrate foods contain fibre, vitamins and minerals, and they take longer to digest, which means they have less of an immediate impact on blood sugar, causing it to rise more slowly.

Table 3.1: Categories of dietary carbohydrates and their digestive process in the human gut

Class	Number of units	Name of carbohydrate	Food source	Site of digestion	Absorbed as
Simple carbohydrates					
-Monosaccharide	1	Sucrose, maltose, lactose	Sugar Milk Fruit	Small intestine	Glucose, Fructose, Galactose
-Disaccharide	2				
Complex carbohydrate					
-Oligosaccharide	3-9	Starch, Cellulose, Pectin, Dietary Fibre	Grains, Beans, Vegetables	Small intestine	Glucose
-Polysaccharide	>9			Large intestine	Short-chain fatty acid

By this classification, grains and beans contain complex carbohydrates as starches (long chains of glucose) encapsulated within another complex carbohydrate cellulose and fibre. Your body does not have adequate enzymes to break down the fibre. For this reason, it passes into the colon and ferments for further digestion and absorption. This process is time-consuming; hence the glucose rises slowly, blood sugar levels remain stable, and fullness lasts longer.

Figure 3.3: Pyramid of carbohydrate structure

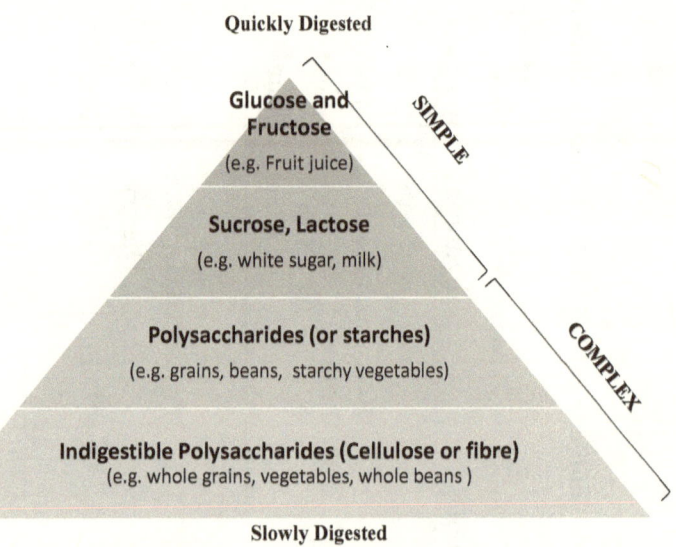

Adapted from Holford P, 2005 New optimum Nutrition Bible

You may have heard your healthcare provider asking you to avoid refined carbohydrates. What does this mean?

Recent years have seen carbohydrates getting a bad rap, mainly because people associate them with white bread, pasta, and rice, as well as sweetened yoghurts and juices. It is true that not all carbohydrates are bad, but when carbs are refined, many beneficial nutrients are lost. So, it is important to understand the difference between refined and unrefined carbohydrates.

Refined Vs Unrefined Carbohydrates

Refined carbohydrates are referred to as 'simple' carbohydrates, including sugars (e.g., glucose, fructose, sucrose) or/and anything made from starch-based grains (wheat, rice) that have had the fibrous wheat germ and bran removed (refined grains).

Refined carbohydrates = simple carbohydrates and/or refined grains.

Increased consumption of refined carbohydrates creates a cascade of adverse effects on your liver, causing liver insulin resistance, fatty liver, increased triglyceride, and LDL-cholesterol as well as increasing the fat accumulation in the muscle cells and adipose tissue.

Excessive consumption of starch-based foods, like refined grains, has been shown to increase insulin resistance and the risk of type 2 diabetes.[34] Research strongly suggests consumption of simple carbohydrates not only creates an increased risk for type 2 diabetes but also heart disease and pancreatic cancers.[35]

Examples of refined carbohydrates are white rice, refined flour, refined white sugar, corn syrup, fruit juice concentrates, 'white' noodles, 'white' pasta, bread, and breakfast cereals.

Unrefined carbohydrates include whole grains, burghul, oats, whole beans, lentils, potatoes especially with skins and sweet potato, and anything made with these (wholewheat pasta, bread, noodles and brown rice).

Refined Grains Vs. Whole Grains

Walking through the aisles of the supermarket and seeing all the different types of grains with claims of being healthy, high fibre, low glycemic index, unpolished, brown bread can be overwhelming. There are so many choices for today's shoppers, but it can be difficult to know whether that oven-fresh loaf is packed with whole grains and is also low in added sugars and sodium. So, how do you choose? How do you know if the grain is whole or refined?

Well, "refined grains" are grains that are highly mechanically broken or altered with the addition of artificial chemicals and sugars. Their natural nutrients, such as fibre, vitamins, and minerals, have been reduced or eliminated.

Grains like wheat, rice, corn, and oats are the major sources of carbohydrates in our diet. The problem is we don't consume them as they are produced on the farm. They are processed in a way that makes them unrecognisable from their original form. For instance, the physical appearance of noodles and cornflakes is far from wheat kernels and corncobs.

Figure 3.4: Structure of Whole Grain and Refined Grain

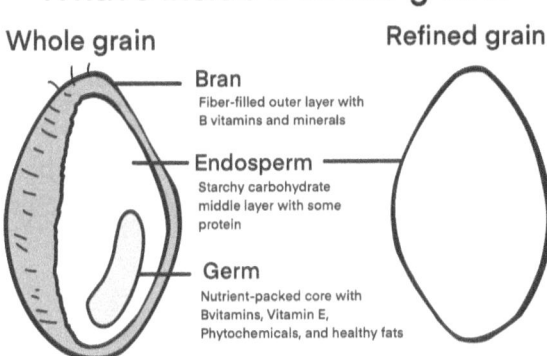

In a nutshell, when a whole grain is mechanically milled to strip the bran and germ portions, leaving the endosperm (mostly starch) part of the seed, this is called refined grain. In other words, refined grains are mostly starch, devoid of essential fibre, vitamins, minerals, and antioxidants.

You might be asking, why do they do that? Well, the answer is simple, to increase the shelf life and therefore the monetary value. Refined and processed foods are less nutritious not just to us but also to the pests that compete with us for their food to survive. Processed foods are easier and quicker to prepare, and easier to digest (the tough barrier of fibre is lost, the release of sugar becomes easier) and they can 'taste' better and last longer.

What is also true is that refined grains and their products made from flour are metabolised and absorbed quickly, resulting in a sharp spike in glucose in your blood within 1-2 hours. Your body doesn't need to work hard breaking down the food structure matrix and complex glucose chains as the food factories' mechanical processing has already done that and the food is now ready to be quickly absorbed.

There is nothing nutritionally valuable about this "appealing" white flour made from wheat, corn, or other grains. It is depleted of all nutrients except for starch which can be broken down into glucose. For this reason, when you switch from highly processed bread to whole grain meal, you see a dramatic improvement in your post-meal glucose spikes.

In direct contrast "whole grains" are either present in their whole form or ground into flour while retaining all parts of the seed (bran, germ, and endosperm). These grains are better sources of fibre and other important nutrients, such as B vitamins, iron, folate, selenium, potassium, and magnesium. Whole grains are either single foods, such as brown rice and popcorn, or ingredients in products, such as buckwheat in pancakes or whole-wheat flour in bread.

The most commonly consumed whole grains include brown rice, wild rice, wheat, oats (oatmeal), corn, barley, buckwheat, bulgur (cracked wheat), amaranth, sorghum, rye, quinoa, and freekeh based on different geographical areas.

Research Evidence

A study published in the British Medical Journal from Harvard University followed 18,000 healthy participants for 30 years, and reported that higher consumption of total whole grains like whole grain breakfast cereal, oatmeal, dark bread, brown rice, added bran, and wheat germ, could be strongly linked to reducing the risk of type 2 diabetes. The authors suggested consuming at least two or more servings of whole grains every day (1 serving = 1/2 cup cooked grain or whole-grain pasta or one slice whole grain bread) to prevent type 2 diabetes.[36]

In fact, a comprehensive overview of 53 reviews suggests that an increase of 30 gm (1 portion) of whole grain every day could reduce the risk of type 2 diabetes by 13%. High intake of whole grain and cereal fibre has been associated with greater insulin sensitivity, lower fasting insulin concentrations, and lower concentrations of inflammatory markers such as C-reactive protein.

On the contrary, the risk of type 2 diabetes increases by 26% with every serving of sugar-sweetened beverages (non-diet soft drinks/sodas, flavoured juice drinks, sports drinks, energy drinks).[37]

Another thorough review of 243 research studies published in the Lancet has indicated that a daily intake of 30 grams of dietary fibre from whole grains could prevent early death due to causes like diabetes, heart disease, and colorectal cancers. The research investigated naturally occurring fibre in whole foods, not isolated fibre added to foods or supplements.[38]

To consume 30 g of fibre a day, you need to eat whole grains, vegetables and fruits at every meal. If you replace one slice of white bread with a slice of whole grain bread, you will gain around 2-3 grams. Choose whole grains like burghul, unpolished brown rice, quinoa, and millets like ragi, jowar, or carly, in preference to refined grains. And ensuring you have at least 5 portions of veg and fruit a day will help you reach the optimum fibre intake.

Whole foods rich in fibre retain much of their structure in the gut, which helps to promote satiety and weight control. Furthermore, fibre in the gut reduces cholesterol absorption and slows blood sugar rises after eating.

How do I read the food label for complex carbohydrates?

Unfortunately, when you look in the supermarket for whole grain packaged products, you won't find whole-grain servings listed on the 'nutrition facts' panel. But there are a few reliable ways to identify whole-grain foods.

Consider these points when you're standing in the grains and bread aisle.

i. **Don't rely on front-of-the-package marketing.**

Just because the package shows the image of a beautiful wheat field does not necessarily mean its contents are made with whole grain. Remember that many products labelled "whole grain" actually contain a mix of whole and refined grains. The food-labelling laws do not regulate the use of the words 'whole grain.' In fact, 'whole grain' products can contain as little as 15 percent to as much as 85 percent whole grains. A whole range of words like "whole grain," "whole wheat flour," "multigrain," "stone ground," "cracked wheat," "wheat," "double fibre," "7 grain," "enriched," "fortified," or "made with whole grains" may be mostly enriched white flour.

ii. **Do not assume that darker is better.**

A darker loaf of bread does not necessarily mean it's made with whole grains—it could simply contain colourings like molasses, malt or caramel or such a small amount of whole wheat that its nutritional benefits are no different from white bread. In fact, "brown bread" can contain even more sugar than its white counterparts.

According to the USDA, one slice of generic brown bread contains 3 grams of sugar, while one slice of the white variety contains 1.64 grams. Brown bread calories can also be higher—110 per slice versus 77 for the white version.[39] However, this information varies by brand. Instead, move on to read the food labels for more accurate information.

iii. **Check the Ingredients List**

Start by checking the list of ingredients to see if the whole grain is listed in the first three ingredients. The relative amount of whole grain in the food can be gauged by the order of placement of the grain in the ingredients list. The whole grain should be the first ingredient or the second ingredient, after water. Choose foods that list "whole" or "whole grain" before the grain's name, such as whole rye flour, whole wheat flour, or whole buckwheat.

Where possible, get your bread from a baker that you can ask and trust the ingredients. Mass-produced bread is never going to be as healthy as bread made freshly on a daily basis.

        Whole grain   Refined grain

> Example: **whole wheat flour, enriched wheat flour** (Flour, Niacin, Riboflavin, Folic acid), corn syrup, Vegetable oils (canola), sodium ascorbate (vitamin C), mixed tocopherol (vitamin E), BHT.
>
> **When choosing bread, also consider the below points**
>
> 1. **Too much sugar?** Look for other sources of added sugars like "no high fructose corn syrup," "molasses," "cane sugar," or "honey." Some breads have 4 grams or more per slice, but 2 grams or less is best.
> 2. **Watch the sodium count.** Bread without salt can taste bland, but some have more than is required. Choose those with about 150 mg or less a slice.
> 3. **How much fibre?** About 2 or 3 grams a slice could mean it has sufficient fibre.
> 4. **Nuts and seeds are good, too.** As long as the bread you choose is all whole grain, getting one with nuts and seeds can mean nice extras: healthy fats and a bit more fibre.

It is recommended that *at least* **half of the grains you eat should be whole grains.**[40] I would like to draw your attention to "at least," and recommend that you aim for as near to 100% as possible. 50% or more will give you better glucose control and lower inflammation, lesser heart problems, and better gut health, which will prevent you from all sorts of chronic diseases like high blood pressure, diabetes, heart disease, cancer, and obesity.

If you are not comfortable with the texture of the whole grain products, try making bread by adding fibre or protein-rich ingredients like pea flour, lentils, soy flour, millet flour, or high-fibre vegetables like spinach, fenugreek, spring onion, carrot, sweet potato.

If you want to go gluten-free, choose naturally gluten-free grains such as unprocessed rice, quinoa, sorghum, buckwheat, legume, and amaranth.

Fruit and Vegetable Carbohydrates

Fruits and vegetables are an excellent package of sugar (glucose, fructose, sucrose), fibre, vitamins, minerals, and phytochemicals. For example, a medium apple has 10.7 grams of fructose, 4.4 grams of glucose, 3.8 grams of sucrose and 4.4 grams of dietary fibre.

Vegetables also contain these sugars in addition to starches. We can divide them into starchy (potato, sweet potato, peas, pumpkin) and non-starchy vegetables (green leafy vegetables, eggplant, broccoli, gourds).

Although they contain sugars and starch, you don't need to worry as much about sugars from fruits and vegetables, as these are packaged along with other essential nutrients and, most importantly, fibre and phytonutrients (plant-based nutrients like antioxidants, flavonoids, plant sterols, isoflavones).

Common serving sizes of fruits and vegetables contain 1–5 g of fibre. These fibres, like starches, are made mostly of many sugar units bonded together (we have discussed earlier the beads strung together).

The digestive enzymes cannot break down these bonds, so they pass relatively intact through the large intestine, contrary to starch molecules which are broken down in the small intestine into glucose molecules. The fibre reaches the large intestine and can be fermented by the colonic microflora to form short-chain fatty acids that are beneficial to health.

This is the reason why fresh fruits do not raise blood glucose as much as fruit juice, as the juices are devoid of fibre. For example, an apple with skin contains 2.4 to 4.4 gm of fibre, and 1 cup of apple juice gives 0.25 gm of total dietary fibre.[41]

Fruits and vegetables usually contain a mix of the two types of fibre—soluble and insoluble—each playing different roles in the body. The soluble fibre dissolves in water to form a gel-like material. It can help lower blood cholesterol and glucose levels. Citrus fruits, apples, brussels sprouts, asparagus, sweet potatoes, turnips, apricots, and mangoes are among the better fruit and vegetable sources of soluble fibre.

While insoluble fibre promotes the movement of material through your digestive system and increases stool bulk, it can be of benefit to those who struggle with constipation or irregular stools. Peas, turnips, kale, raspberries, and pears contain relatively high amounts of insoluble fibre.

Milk Carbohydrates

Carbohydrates take the form of lactose (glucose plus galactose) in milk. Lactose is a natural sugar, giving a sweet flavour to plain milk and yoghurt. Lactose is converted to lactic acid in the process of making cheese. Therefore, cheese has much less lactose when compared to milk. For instance, most contain less than 2 grams per serving (1 ounce), which is far less than the 12 to 13 grams of lactose you get in one serving (1 cup) of milk.

Fat reduction does not affect the carbohydrate content of milk. A cup of full-fat milk, low-fat milk, or fat-free milk contains the same amount of carbohydrate as lactose (12 grams). However, some non-dairy milk choices, like almond milk and soy milk, contain less than 5 grams of carbohydrates in one cup.

Carbohydrates and Digestion

The digestive fate of a particular carbohydrate depends on the chemical and physical structure of the carbohydrate. When you eat carbohydrates, they are broken down by a battery of hydrolytic enzymes starting from the mouth (alpha-amylase) to the pancreas (pancreatic-amylase) and eventually in the intestine brush border lining (lactase, sucrase, and maltase).

These carbohydrates are broken down into one bead monosaccharide (G, Gl, F) for absorption into the blood circulation to be transported via the portal vein to the liver. The ones that are not broken down by these enzymes are digested by the process of fermentation in the large bowel (colon) to form short-chain fatty acids.

The rate of uptake of glucose (and other sugars) from the gut depends on many factors. Food particle size, intact cell walls, level of food processing, mixed with fat and protein, chewing of food, consistency of food, rate of emptying by the stomach (gastric emptying), to name a few.

Most of the fructose and galactose molecules are absorbed by the liver through specific receptors and metabolised (changed into a form that can be used by the body). The glucose enters the liver cells (through GLUT 2 transporter channels) and burns in furnaces (mitochondria) to release energy (Adenosine triphosphate-ATP). This process is dependent on insulin.

The excess glucose is then stored as glycogen (stockpile of glucose), or pushed into circulation for use by muscle, adipose, and other tissues. Similar to the liver, a muscle can either use glucose to burn as immediate energy or stack it up as glycogen and fatty acid for later use for physical activities or when at rest. (Discussed in detail in Chapter 2).

However, only your liver and muscle can store large quantities of glycogen. The reason why the liver stocks glucose as glycogen is to maintain the supply of glucose to the brain, as it needs a continuous glucose uptake for its functioning (glucose is the main source of energy for the brain).

This is a reason why, when you restrict carbohydrates in your diet, your brain is forced to adapt to a new fuel called ketone bodies (produced by the liver as an emergency backup fuel). Other than a steady supply of glucose to the brain, glycogen also feeds glucose to the demands of other activities like fasting, exercising, or sleeping through a process called gluconeogenesis.

If you have diabetes, gluconeogenesis is often increased, which leads to the liver producing an unnecessary amount of sugar at night, which gives elevated fasting glucose values in the morning. This is partly because the liver is insulin resistant.

The insulin released after eating carbohydrates does not depend only on the starch/glucose in the meal or the rate at which food is moving out of the gut (gastric emptying) but also by the cellular structure of the food particles. These effects may be mediated through a battery of hormones (Ghrelin, peptide YY, Glucagon like peptide-1, cholecystokinin) that are released by the gut which control your feeling of fullness and hunger.[42]

This process seems quite straightforward, but there are several feedback mechanisms and hormones that synchronise this process, and the hormone that is released, i.e. "insulin."

Metabolism of carbohydrates that do not release glucose (non-glycaemic)

Whole grains, fruits, and vegetables contain complex carbohydrates that can't be absorbed in the small intestine and enter the large bowel, where bacteria are able to partially or completely break them down into simpler carbohydrates.

How do we know which food is digested to release glucose and which one ferments in the colon? Well, this depends on the physical and chemical structure of the food item. Some foods are partially digested and absorbed in the small intestine, like rice/wheat, where starch (amylase/amylopectin) is potentially digested in the small intestine.

However, if starch is trapped inside an intact cell wall, it remains inaccessible to the intestinal enzymes and moves to the colon for fermentation. This is a reason we see a plateau peak after someone eats whole grain bread compared to a sharp glucose spike after eating highly processed refined flour bread.

In addition, fruits change their digestion ability with the stage of ripeness. For instance, a ripe banana digests as sugar, whereas an unripe banana is partially digested as sugar, and the unripe starch (resistant starch) is further fermented.

Carbohydrates which reach the large colon ferment to release short-chain fatty acids (SCFA) like acetic, propionic, and butyric acids. Most of these short-chain fatty acids are absorbed and provide up to 10% of the body's energy supply.[43]

These SCFAs in the blood circulation perform important roles as they affect glucose storage in the muscle, liver, and fat. Acetate reaches the brain and decreases appetite which decreases food consumption, promotes immunity, prevents inflammatory diseases and enhances the gut barrier to prevent inflammatory diseases caused by invading bacteria.

These functions are also likely to contribute to the suppression of autoimmune lymphocytes and type 1 diabetes; however, this is not conclusive yet.

Glycemic Index Vs. Glycemic Load
Glycemic index

So, if carbohydrates raise blood glucose levels and some cause blood sugar levels to rise rapidly, while others cause them to rise moderately or slowly, you might be wondering if there is a way to find out which is which?

An easy way to explain how carbohydrate-rich foods affect blood sugar was developed by Jenkins in 1981: the "Glycemic Index" (GI).[44]

The glycemic index ranks carbohydrates on a scale of 0 to 100 depending on how quickly and how high they raise blood glucose levels after eating. Foods with a high GI, like white bread, are rapidly digested and cause substantial fluctuations in blood glucose. Foods with a low GI, like whole grains, are digested more slowly, prompting a more gradual rise in blood glucose. Low-glycemic foods have a GI of 55 or less, medium-level foods have a GI of 56-69, and high-glycemic foods have a GI of 70-100.

There are many factors that can affect a food's glycemic index, for instance:

Processing and cooking increase the GI as it alters the natural form and size of food particles. Whole grains have a lower GI than refined grains as they are devoid of bran and germ (as discussed before). Finely ground grain is more rapidly digested than coarsely ground grain (whole meal flour vs. refined wheat flour). Liquid foods will have a higher GI compared to solid foods due to ease of digestion and absorption. For example, the GI of fresh orange is 40, while that of fresh orange juice is 48.

Foods high in fat, protein, and fibre generally have a lower glycaemic response, since they slow stomach emptying and digestion, resulting in a lower GI. The ripeness of food affects its GI too. An unripe banana may have a GI of 30, while that of a ripe banana is 51.

Nonetheless, this is not the whole story, as we rarely eat just one sort of food in a meal. For a snack, you may just have a banana, but for lunch, you wouldn't just eat a bowl of pasta. You would cook it with sauce or vegetables, perhaps some protein and may have a bowl of salad on the side. In this case, the blood glucose after a meal is a consequence of the mixed meal rather than from just one food item.

Combining low GI and high GI foods in a meal has the effect of 'averaging' the GI. You can reduce the GI of your meals by mixing low and medium GI foods together so that the average GI of each meal is reduced. For instance, the overall effect of rice on blood glucose will be reduced when large quantities of non-starchy vegetables are added to it.

Figure 3.5: Post-meal glucose response on a low GI and high GI food

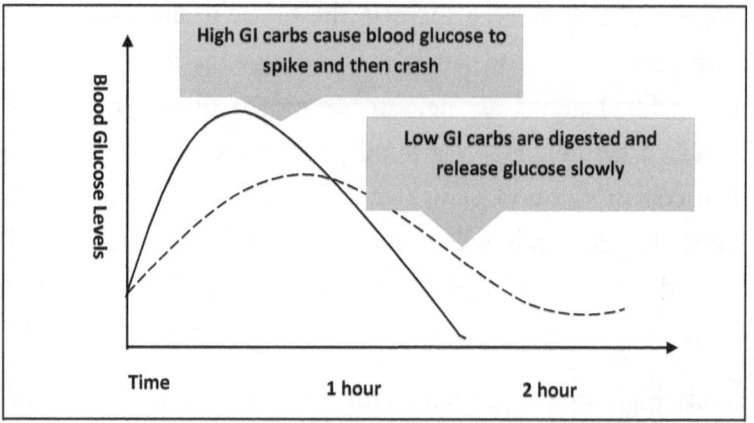

Glycemic Load

Simple carbohydrates spike blood glucose levels and have a higher glycemic index. In addition to the type of carbohydrates, blood glucose spikes are also influenced by the quantity of carbohydrate, and GI does not account for this. For example, even though pasta has a low GI, a large serving can still cause blood glucose levels to rise more rapidly than a smaller serving.

As a result of this shortcoming in GI, researchers developed another index that takes into account both the amount and type of carbohydrates and their effect on blood glucose levels. This measure is called the glycemic load (GL). The GL builds on GI, as it takes into consideration both the GI of the food and the amount of carbohydrates in a portion.

A food's glycemic load is determined by multiplying its glycemic index by the amount of carbohydrates the food contains. In general, a glycemic load score of 20 or more is high, 11 to 19 is medium, and 10 or under is low.

A large number of studies have concluded that people who consumed lower-glycemic load diets were at a lower risk of developing type 2 diabetes and coronary heart disease than those who ate a diet of higher-glycemic load foods.[45, 46]

A number of resources are available on the internet and apps that give you the charts of GI and GL.

Dietary Fat 101

In the early 1980s, the U.S. Department of Agriculture recommended avoiding all three main categories of fat i.e., unsaturated fats, saturated fats and trans fats. The low-fat diet became a craze, and lots of "low-fat" items flooded the shelves of grocery stores.

The problem was that many of these products replaced the fat with refined sugars and sugar substitutes, knocking out any health benefits. All dietary fats were deemed bad, despite the fact that fat is an essential nutrient and has protective properties too.

The dietary guidelines and published research on the subject have taken enough twists and turns to leave many people confused.

So, if you're confused about the health effects of fats, you are not alone. You've probably read headlines in the paper, claiming that fats are killing us all only to find another week later, claiming that they're actually really healthy for us.

We cannot ignore the importance of dietary fats in our diet. These food sources provide us with energy and essential fatty acids (your body cannot make these fatty acids, but they are crucial for health) such as omega 3 and omega 6. And of course, adding some amount of fat makes your food taste great.

No doubt, carbohydrates get all the attention when we talk about controlling your blood glucose. However, dietary fat also affects blood glucose. Both the quantity and the quality of fat affect your blood glucose – and not all fat is equal!

There is only one thing that is equal about all fats and oils: they are all equicaloric (equal calories). In other words, 1 gm of coconut oil/olive oil/butter/sunflower oil/almond oil or any other oil/fat gives you about 9 kcal. One tsp (5gm) of olive oil, butter, sunflower oil, or sesame oil gives you 45 kcal. The difference is not in the calories they provide but the type of fatty acid they are made of, as this determines the quality of fat and the impact they have on your health.

When we talk about fat, it's also important to understand that although we use this term synonymously when referring to fat in the human body and in dietary sources, they are not the same.

In this next section, I will be discussing dietary fats (fats found in food sources, both plant and animal) and their impact on blood glucose.

Like carbohydrates, dietary fats are divided into simple and complex, plant vs. animal, liquid vs. solid fats, and saturated vs. unsaturated. We will look specifically at the classification of fats based on their significant impact on your health.

You might think a nut would be a good source of unsaturated fats, but it also contains a small amount of saturated fat. An egg combines saturated fats, unsaturated fats, and cholesterol.

Do all fats in our diet pose a health risk? Are some fats terrible and others a cure-all?

Let's try to clear this up.

Saturated Fat

Saturated fats are solid at room temperature and are commonly found in animal products, meat, egg, chicken, fish, and meat products (sausage, bacon, beef, hamburger), whole milk, butter, cheese, and dairy desserts. Also found in certain plant foods like coconut oil, palm oil, and cocoa butter.

We have discussed in detail in Chapter 2 the role of dietary fat in insulin resistance. However, we did not dig into the type of fat. As early as 1927, it was reported that increased fat consumption delays the process of blood sugars going into the cells, which means sugars hang around longer in the bloodstream. Later, several animal and human studies showed that a high intake of saturated fat is associated with insulin resistance and the development of type 2 diabetes.[47]

Are saturated fatty acids good, bad, or just fine?

The answer to this question is not simple, as we have a robust debate on whether saturated fat improves or deteriorates diabetes health. The advocates of a low-carbohydrate diet, ketogenic diets, and paleo diet argue that although these diets are high in saturated fat, they improve glucose control as it lacks carbohydrates (the reason for the glucose spike). On the contrary, the supporters of low-fat, plant-based diets insist that saturated fat increases insulin resistance and promotes heart diseases and cancer.

To put this argument in perspective, you need to understand the strength of research studies and the study's outcome, which can be tricky to comprehend. I have tried to explain in simple, understandable language here.

There is enough evidence to state that weight loss induced by a low-calorie diet reduces insulin resistance and hence, improves blood glucose absorption. And this low-calorie diet could be a low-fat diet, low-carbohydrate diet, very low-calorie diet, high-fat diet, or any other diet with different proportions of these macronutrients (fat, carbohydrate, protein). Indicating that the improvement is attributed to weight loss rather than the ratio of macronutrients.

The high-fat diets are mostly high in saturated fat, and these diets may result in an excellent blood glucose level and lower HbA1c values, but this improvement comes at the expense of significantly increased insulin resistance, which I have described earlier as the known reason for increased heart disease, cancer, Alzheimer's and premature death.

Most of the research studies that show the benefits of high saturated fat in terms of weight loss or glucose control are short-term treatments (less than one year). The long-term studies do not show the same benefits. On the contrary, long-term adherence to this sort of diet has shown an increase in the overall risk of chronic diseases and premature death.[48]

Here's the thing. We do not eat nutrients, we eat food. And all natural food items are a combination of nutrients and non-nutrients in specific proportions. Hence, when we say a high-fat diet or low-carbohydrate diet, we are only considering the major nutrient but failing to recognise the compound effect of other nutrients' presence or absence.

It is all about substitution. If you remove one type of fat, what are you replacing it with? Cutting back on saturated fat can be good for health if people replace saturated fat with good fats, especially polyunsaturated fats. If you remove saturated fat and replace it with refined carbohydrates, there will be a detrimental effect.

So, we need to think about food quality including food sources and dietary patterns rather than nutrients alone.

Altering your diet for a short duration of a few weeks and having large amounts of saturated fat (more than 10 grams per day) are reported to increase insulin resistance, which could last for days or months after stopping it, depending on the amount of saturated fat and frequency of consuming it. And a meal high in saturated fat could increase saturated fatty acids within the liver and contribute to hepatic insulin resistance (the liver refusing to open the doors for glucose to enter).

It can also cause a binding affinity of cell membranes to insulin, increased inflammatory cytokines leading to low-grade inflammation, and direct inhibition of the action of insulin.

Other than insulin resistance, diets high in saturated fat are also dangerous for nasty fatty liver disease. The excessive fatty acids in the liver not only damage the optimum functions of the liver but as we have said, lead to an advanced state of insulin resistance and liver inflammation.

How do you know that there are these detrimental changes in the liver? This is reflected in increased fasting blood glucose, increased triglycerides, and increased LDL-cholesterol values in your blood test reports. And the signs of fat deposition in the liver are reflected in elevated liver enzyme (ALT, AST, GGT, etc.) tests.

Unsaturated Fat

Unsaturated fats are liquid at room temperature. Contrary to saturated fats, unsaturated fat offers protection against insulin resistance when consumed in small quantities. They also improve blood cholesterol, ease inflammation and stabilise heart rhythms, to name a few important functions. These fats are predominantly found in plant foods like vegetable oils, seeds, and nuts.

Unsaturated fats hold two types of "good" fatty acids: monounsaturated fatty acids (MUFA) and polyunsaturated fatty acids (PUFA).

The MUFA are highly available in avocado, canola oil, olives, olive oil, safflower oil, and nuts. The MUFA can also be made by your body if you are not consuming them in food, whereas the PUFA are considered essential because your body cannot make them by itself but has to absorb them from food.

Both fatty acids help in reducing LDL cholesterol, an important marker of heart health. However, PUFA has a greater association with a reduced risk of diabetes. This beneficial effect is derived from the specific PUFA, omega-3, and omega-6.

Omega-3 Fatty Acids

You will have heard that fish is a good source of this magic fat which will prevent you from having a heart attack, but it isn't the fish that creates the magic. Taking a few steps backward, fish get the Omegas originally from green plants, specifically algae. Hence, the animal sources fishes like salmon, mackerel, and sardine, and the plant sources like flax seeds, chia seeds, walnut, purslane, seaweed, and algae are all high in this magic fatty acid.

When you are looking for supplements of omega-3-fatty acids, you may come across these complicated scientific words. There are three types of omega-3 fats based on their sources. Fish contain Eicosapentaenoic acid (EPA) and Docosahexaenoic acid (DHA) which is referred to as "marine omega-3." On the other hand, plants sources contain alpha-linolenic acid (ALA).

The omega-3 fatty acids are an integral part of cell membranes throughout the body and affect the function of the cell receptors in these membranes. They provide the starting point for making hormones that regulate blood clotting, contraction and relaxation of artery walls, glucose metabolism and calming of inflammation.

Omega-6 Fatty Acids

Often found in nuts and seeds and eventually in oils drawn from these sources. These include sunflower oil, soybean oil, almond, walnut, corn, and cashews.

Omega-6 fats are involved in the rigidity of cell walls, clotting of blood, and the triggering of inflammatory response.

The interesting fact is that these two fatty acids compete with each other to execute their respective role in the body. Hence, making the ratio of consumption between them very crucial for your health. In other words, too much omega-6 rich vegetable oil consumption may be as dangerous as too little omega-3 rich fish, flax seeds, or chia seeds for inflammation and protection of heart health.

The Art of Balance Through Substitution-Research Evidence

Dutch researchers conducted an analysis of 60 trials that examined the effects of carbohydrates and various fats on blood lipid levels. When polyunsaturated and monounsaturated fats were substituted for carbohydrates in trials, these good fats decreased levels of harmful LDL-cholesterol and increased protective HDL cholesterol.[49]

An interesting study published in the New England of Medicine (DIRECT trial) pared equal calorie low-fat, low-carbohydrate and Mediterranean diets for two years and concluded that people with diabetes have the best results with insulin resistance and glucose spike (HbA1c) with the Mediterranean diet (50 percent from whole carbohydrate-high dietary fibre, high monounsaturated to saturated fat ratio). This emphasises the need for optimum substitution of fats as a key factor not only for glucose control but also for heart health.[50]

Another impressive prospective cohort of the Nurse's Health Study (34 years follow-up) and Health Professionals' Follow-Up Study (28 years follow-up) concluded that in an isocaloric model (Isocaloric means having the same daily calories, but the proportion of fats, carbohydrates and protein may vary), replacing just 2% of calories from saturated fatty acids with PUFAs, is associated with 13% lower death due to heart diseases. This is staggering, 2% of calories represents just 40 calories out of an average 2,000 calories per day.[51]

The overarching message was that when it comes to the health values of various fats, it's about substitution. Reducing saturated fat can be good for health if you replace that with good fats, especially polyunsaturated fats. Moreover, we need to consider food as a whole, including food sources and dietary patterns, rather than nutrients alone.

Trans Fat

Trans fats are produced when liquid oil is made into solid fat—a process called hydrogenation. Although a very small quantity is also found in beef, pork, lamb, butter, and milk, and is formed by bacteria in the stomachs of cattle, sheep, and goats; this is not a cause for concern in its natural form. Most trans fats are artificially made and come from processed foods.

Trans fats are the worst type of fat for the heart, blood vessels, and the rest of the body because they raise bad LDL-cholesterol and lower good HDL-cholesterol, create inflammation, and contribute to insulin resistance. These trans fats are hidden everywhere in ultra-processed foods (discussed in Chapter 6).

A Harvard study involving over 140,000 participants found that for every 2 percent increase in daily calories from trans-fat, the risk of coronary heart disease increases by 23 percent.[52]

Trans fats are listed on the Nutrition Facts label, making it easier to identify these foods. However, keep in mind that less than 0.5 grams is claimed as 0% trans-fat on the label. To avoid as much trans-fat as possible, you should read the ingredients list on food labels. Look for words like hydrogenated oil or partially hydrogenated oil. Avoid foods where liquid oil is listed first on the ingredients list.

The most common sources of trans fats are ultra-processed foods like fast food, crackers, and chips, as well as baked goods like muffins, cookies, and cakes or partially hydrogenated oils such as margarine and shortening that are semi-soft. These are used to increase the shelf-life of foods as well as their flavour stability.

Dietary Cholesterol

Cholesterol is the raw material that makes a lot of vital components in the animal and human body, for instance, certain hormones, vitamin D, and cell membranes. Dietary cholesterol comes only from animal products like meat, chicken, fish, and dairy. Animal fat is different from plant-based fat. It is usually high in saturated fat and found as white strips in meat cuts or greasy residue coming out of grilled fish. You can feel the animal fat, but cholesterol is a microscopic ingredient embedded in the cells of all animal products in different proportions. Some foods are enlisted in the table below.

Table 3.2 Dietary cholesterol in food items

Food Products	Portion	Cholesterol (mg)
Milk (non-fat)	1 cup	5
Milk (low-fat)	1 cup	20
Milk (whole)	1 cup	34
Cheddar Cheese	1 cup	131
Butter	1 tsp	11
Egg	1 large	186
Shrimp	3 ½ oz	194
Chicken (no skin)	3 ½ oz/100gm	85
Lamb (foreshank)	3 ½ oz	106
Salmon	3 ½ oz	63
Pinto beans	1/2 cup	0
Vegetable Oils	1 tsp	0

Reference: United States Department of Agriculture (USDA, 2018)[53]

The American Diabetes Association recommends that people with diabetes should consume less than 300 mg of cholesterol per day.

Why is consuming excessive saturated fats and dietary cholesterol a risk for heart disease?

To understand the influence of dietary fats on your heart, you need to start with lipids - another word for blood fats. Fats are part of every cell in your body.

Cholesterol is an important part of cell membranes, certain vitamins, and hormones, while triglycerides are stored fats that keep you warm, protect the body's organs, and reserve a source of fuel. These triglycerides are made up of building blocks—fatty acids. When the sources of glucose deplete, these fatty acids are used for energy.

Cholesterol and triglycerides travel through your body in the blood for various vital functions. However, they need a carrier to take them from one destination to the other. Just like raw material is sent to factories in trucks, these particles are carried by lipoproteins (lipo means fat).

The fact that they (the fats) need a special means of transport in the blood is due to the fact that the blood is an aqueous solution and fat is not, therefore some kind of transport mechanism is needed.

You might hear your physician saying, "Your low-density lipoprotein cholesterol (LDL-Cholesterol) is high, or high-density lipoprotein cholesterol (HDL-Cholesterol) is low."

What does that mean and how do they influence your heart health?

There are two types of lipoproteins that help in the transportation of cholesterol.

1. Low-density lipoprotein (LDL) cholesterol: These particles carry cholesterol to the tissues, and in the process, they often get stuck in the lining of blood vessel walls. As a consequence, they spark the formation of raised bumps called plaques, which are similar to scars on the artery linings. This can lead to atherosclerosis or hardening of the arteries.
   Why is it dangerous to have these plaques?
   This is dangerous because plaques are fragile. They crack and cause blood clots for damage control. The job of a blood clot is to stop blood flow. If this happens in the artery carrying blood to the heart though, it can cause a heart attack, and if this happens in the brain, it can cause a stroke. This is the reason that LDL cholesterol is considered "bad" cholesterol.
2. High-density lipoprotein (HDL) cholesterol: These lipoproteins pull cholesterol out of the tissues and return it to the liver. Since it is involved in reverse cholesterol transport, it is considered your "good" cholesterol.

Meanwhile, the triglycerides, cholesterol, and other fats are carried by another lipoprotein called very-low-density lipoprotein (VLDL). VLDL drops off triglycerides and other fats in the fat tissue and then becomes LDL.

People with diabetes often have high LDL and VLDL levels and low HDL levels, which means more bad and less good cholesterol, hence increasing the risk of heart disease.

The solution to this problem is to reduce the circulating cholesterol particles in the bloodstream. So, how can you do that?

Keto Diets and Cholesterol

Sometimes referred to as the "keto" diet, the ketogenic diet is a strict eating pattern high in fat, moderate in protein, and low in carbohydrates.[54] Although there are many different forms of the ketogenic diet, clinical trials and popular versions of this diet generally restrict daily carbohydrate consumption below 50 grams, primarily from non-starchy vegetables, and emphasize 70-80% fat, 10-20% protein, and 5-10% carbohydrates, of total daily calories.[55]

Many people ask me, "If you significantly remove carbohydrates from your meals, do you achieve better post-meal glucose? Should I go on a ketogenic diet?" I will put things in perspective so that you can decide wisely.

The ketogenic diet helps you lose weight, achieve flat post-meal glucose, reduce or eliminate medication, and reduce cholesterol. So, **why don't I recommend this to my patients, especially those that take insulin and have complications of diabetes?** Below are the most important points of consideration before you decide to adopt the keto diet.

i. When you choose a ketogenic diet, most of your fat comes from animal sources like meat, eggs, sausages, butter, cheese, fish, bacon, cream cheese, or chicken. Evidence-based research conducted in large populations repeatedly shows that eating a high proportion of high-fat animal products increases the risk of type 2 diabetes and premature death.[56]

An umbrella review (a review of the reviews, with very strong evidence) reported that consumption of 100 g/day of total or red meat, or 50 g/day of processed meat, was associated with an increased risk of type 2 diabetes by 20% and 30%, respectively. To reduce the risk of diabetes, red meat and processed meat consumption should be restricted. Moderate consumption of dairy foods, milk, and yoghurt is ok; moderate amounts of fish and eggs are also allowed.[57]

ii. Diabetes is often regarded as merely a matter of managing blood glucose levels. But managing blood sugar levels is only one part of the puzzle. To achieve optimum health and prevent complications of diabetes, you need all the nutrients in the right proportions and the right frequency. The lower your carbohydrate intake, the more you are wiping out entire food groups considered to be nutrient-dense and healthy. What's so compelling about the keto diet that you would give up some cornerstones of healthy eating and nutrition? Suppose you were not eating a wide variety of vegetables, fruits, grains, beans, and nuts? In this case, you may be at risk of nutrient deficiencies and depleted of protective phytonutrients, antioxidants, and dietary fibre. Moreover, these nutrients protect against heart diseases and certain cancers.

iii. Another crucial reason is that diabetes is a lifelong condition, so managing your diabetes needs to work within your lifestyle. Restrictive meal plans like keto can be effective short term, but it's not always the right choice long term, because eating a restrictive diet, no matter what the plan, is difficult to sustain. When you resume eating all food groups again, you will likely regain weight and the associated problems again.

In a study conducted from June 2019 to December 2020, Gardner and his team recruited 40 adults with type 2 diabetes or prediabetes to try both the ketogenic diet and the Mediterranean diet. Half the participants started with the ketogenic diet, and the other half started with the Mediterranean diet.

After 12 weeks, the groups switched and tried the other diet for the next 12 weeks. This crossover design allowed participants to act as their own controls. The researchers found that both diets improved blood glucose control, as indicated by similar drops in HbA1c levels (9% on keto and 7% on the Mediterranean).

Weight loss was also similar (8% on keto and 7% on the Mediterranean), as were improvements in fasting insulin and glucose, HDL cholesterol, and the liver enzyme ALT.[58]

The takeaway for people with diabetes or prediabetes was that the less restrictive Mediterranean diet was similarly effective in controlling glucose and likely more sustainable.

"Restricting added sugars and refined grains and emphasising the inclusion of vegetables should be the focus," Gardner said. "There's no reason to restrict heart-healthy, quality carbohydrate foods above and beyond." [58]

Each diet had one other statistically significant benefit: LDL cholesterol increased on the keto diet and decreased on the Mediterranean diet—a point for the Mediterranean. Triglyceride decreased on both diets but dropped more on the keto diet—a point for keto.

Take Home Messages

1. The simple carbohydrates (sugar, honey) raise blood glucose levels quickly, while the complex carbohydrates (grains, beans, vegetables, fruit) take longer to digest, resulting in slower blood sugar rises.
2. Research review suggests an increase of 30 gm (1 portion) of whole grain every day could reduce the risk of type 2 diabetes by 13%.
3. It is recommended that *at least* half of the grains you eat should be whole grains
4. Start cutting back on saturated fat. Your liver uses the fat to make VLDL. The more fat you eat, the more VLDL the liver makes. More VLDL means more LDL cholesterol.
5. Replace saturated fat (animal products as discussed above) with unsaturated fats (polyunsaturated and monounsaturated).
6. Stay away from ultra-processed food that is a source of trans fats and simple carbohydrates.

CHAPTER 4

CONSEQUENCES OF DIABETES: HEART, NERVES, EYES, AND KIDNEYS

*F*or the majority of the 400 million people in the world, managing diabetes will last their entire lifetime. Making it essential for those with diabetes to have the knowledge and resources to effectively manage their condition. The reality is that you could be struggling with daily decisions that will affect blood glucose: when to test, when to eat, how much to eat, when to correct, whether it is safe to exercise, is it safe to fast for long hours and even whether it is safe to work at night.

These are just some immediate questions. I am sure there is an additional layer of scary concerns like, what will happen if I don't control my blood glucose? Will I have a heart attack or stroke? Will I lose my eyesight or be on dialysis? How do I cope with an incurable disease? It would be great to take a break from thinking about diabetes, but diabetes is all day, every day, for a lifetime.

It is important to take good care of diabetes for long-term health. Well-managed diabetes reduces the risk of complications. Managing or reversing the effects of diabetes requires much more effort than just getting your blood glucose under control.

High concentrations of blood glucose over a long period of time may lead to detrimental consequences to your heart, nerve, eyes, and kidney. It can seriously damage your blood vessels and, eventually, your nerves. This means you can lose the sensation in different parts of your body.

Once you've damaged the blood vessels and nerves in one part of your body, you're more likely to develop similar problems in other parts as well. For instance, numbness in the feet due to nerve damage indicates the possibility of an eye problem too.

Fortunately, the consequences of diabetes are not a one-way road. If you have been in poor health or if diabetes has harmed your eyes, heart, kidney, or nerves, revamping your lifestyle choices can have a drastic impact on your well-being and slow down the deterioration.

In this chapter, we will look at how to accomplish effective damage control.

Why Bother About the Consequences of Diabetes?

It may take tremendous effort to get your diabetes under control, but the results will prove to be worth the struggle. Uncontrolled diabetes means your blood glucose levels are too high, even if you're treating it with medications. If you don't make an effort to handle it, you will set yourself up for a host of complications.

Diabetes can take a toll on nearly every organ in your body, including your heart, your eyes, nerves, and kidneys. As the World health organisation reports, diabetes is a major cause of blindness, kidney failure, heart attacks, stroke, and lower limb amputation.[59] You probably already have a good idea of your risk of these problems, as your doctor may have briefed you while discussing blood glucose, blood pressure, and cholesterol levels. I trust they have mentioned to you the need to have optimum control of all the indicators to protect your heart.

Before we take a look at the details of these complications, let's take a step back and learn about the risks themselves. How do you know that you are moving toward complications? What are the indicators that you can monitor to take control of the situation before it escalates?

How do I know if I have an increased risk of complications?

The indicators that show that you are at risk of diabetes-related complications are listed below:

High Blood Pressure (Hypertension)

Hypertension is defined as a systolic blood pressure ≥130 mmHg or a diastolic blood pressure ≥80 mmHg based on an average of ≥2 measurements obtained on ≥2 occasions. Several studies have reported that blood pressure (both systolic and diastolic) variability in people with diabetes is an independent predictor of complications of the heart, nerves, eyes, and kidneys. You should discuss your target blood pressure with your physician as it is determined by your health condition. An optimum blood pressure goal is below 130/80 mmHg.[60]

Smoking

Smoking makes it harder for blood to flow around your body to places like your heart and your feet. If you smoke, then stopping is a key part of reducing your chances of complications. If you find it difficult to quit, start by reducing the number of cigarettes. It can also add to the healing process. Smoking is associated with heart disease, artery disease, foot ulcers, amputation of legs, and retinopathy of the eyes[61] as well as non-diabetes related problems like lung cancer, emphysema and even cataracts and rheumatoid arthritis!

Hba1c (glycated haemoglobin)

Glycaemic control (glucose control) is assessed by the HbA1C measurement. This test shows your average blood sugar level for the past 2 to 3 months. It measures the percentage of blood sugar attached to the haemoglobin molecule, which is the oxygen-carrying protein in red blood cells. The higher your blood glucose levels, the more haemoglobin you'll have with glucose attached.

There is a strong link between high HbA1c readings and the risk of developing diabetes-related complications and them affecting the heart, eye, and nerve health. So good blood glucose is crucial to prevent diabetic complications. The recommended HbA1c goal is less than 7%, however, achieving lower than this may be beneficial if it is achieved safely.[62]

Cholesterol

Diabetes damages the lining of your arteries. This means it's more likely that cholesterol will stick to them, making them narrow or even blocked. If you have diabetes, you will usually have lower levels of HDL (good) cholesterol and higher levels of LDL/non-HDL (bad) cholesterol. This is commonly called 'dyslipidemia' and means your arteries are more likely to become narrow or blocked.

Albumin-to creatinine ratio

A common urine test to check if there is protein in the urine. This is a sign that diabetes has caused kidney damage. If this is the case, your physician will emphasise lowering blood pressure, blood glucose and blood fat levels.

Body weight

Excessive weight (BMI≥30kg/m^2) is a known risk factor for hypertension, dyslipidemia, and poor glycaemic control, thereby increasing the risk of heart disease, stroke, and kidney disease in people with diabetes.

Now, let's look at how and why diabetes damages your health and why it is important to routinely monitor your indicators, as discussed above.

What are the complications of diabetes?

There are two types of complications you may experience.

- Acute (severe and sudden)
- Chronic (starts slowly and long-lasting)

Acute complications

Acute complications include hypoglycaemia and ketoacidosis. These require immediate medical help.

What is hypoglycaemia?

Hypoglycaemia is when your blood glucose falls below the normal range. Glucose in your blood is the main source of energy for your body and brain. When the level of glucose drops, your body can't function properly, leading to symptoms such as:

- Shaking
- Sweating
- Hunger
- Anxiety
- Weakness
- Dizziness
- Lack of concentration
- Speech problems

If you experience these symptoms, you should immediately check your blood glucose. If it is below 70mg/dl (3.9mmol/L) or whatever other benchmark value your doctor has suggested, then you need to seek immediate help. Failure to do so can lead to seizures, unconsciousness, or even death. Those of you taking insulin or any other medication that lowers blood glucose levels should be extra vigilant to detect hypoglycaemia.

What do I do in hypoglycaemia?

Follow the 15-15 rule—have 15 grams of simple carbohydrates to raise your blood sugar and check it after 15 minutes. If it's still below 70 mg/dL, have another serving. Repeat these steps until your blood sugar is at least 70 mg/dL. Once your blood sugar is back to normal, eat a meal or snack, or if it is your mealtime, go ahead and eat to make sure it doesn't lower again.

Sources of simple carbohydrates may include:

1. Glucose tablets (sold in pharmacies),
2. 120ml (1/2 cup) of any fruit juice or regular soft drink, and
3. One tablespoon of sugar and honey mixed in ½ cup water or 5 to 6 pieces of hard candy.

It is often observed that many people in this situation eat as much as they can until they feel better. This can cause blood sugar levels to shoot up too high. Using the step-wise approach of the "15-15 Rule" can help you avoid this, preventing high blood sugar levels.

Young children usually need less than 15 grams of carbs to fix a low blood sugar level. Infants may need 6 grams, toddlers may need 8 grams, and small children may need 10 grams. This needs to be individualised for the patient, so discuss the amount needed with your diabetes team.

Hypoglycaemia in sleep

Sometimes your blood glucose level can drop in the middle of your sleep, and you may wake up with nightmares, soaked with sweat, or feeling unusually tired, confused, or irritable. Check your blood glucose and continue with the 15-15 rule. However, if this happens often, talk to your physician to check if you need to review your medications.

What is diabetic ketoacidosis?

Diabetic ketoacidosis (DKA) is a serious complication of type 1 diabetes. DKA only happens when you don't have enough insulin in your body to process blood sugar into energy, and it can be the first sign in an individual with type 1 diabetes. If this happens, your liver starts to process fat into energy, which releases ketones into the blood. High levels of ketones in the blood can be extremely dangerous.

This is less common in people with type 2 diabetes because insulin levels don't usually drop so low, but it can occur in them as well. Ketoacidosis shouldn't be confused with ketosis, which is harmless. Ketosis can occur as a result of an extremely low carbohydrate diet, known as a ketogenic diet, or from fasting.

How do I know I have diabetic ketoacidosis?

Symptoms of DKA can appear quickly. Early symptoms of DKA can include:

- Frequent urination,
- Extreme thirst or dry mouth,

- High blood sugar levels, also known as hyperglycaemia. and
- High levels of ketones in the urine.

As DKA progresses, more symptoms may appear:
- Nausea or vomiting,
- Abdominal pain,
- Lack of concentration,
- Fruity-smelling breath,
- Flushed face,
- Fatigue or weakness,
- Rapid breathing,
- Dry skin, and
- Loss of consciousness, also known as fainting or syncope.

DKA is a medical emergency. Once it occurs, you should call your local emergency services immediately. If left untreated, DKA can lead to coma or death. If you use insulin, make sure you discuss the risk of DKA with your healthcare team and have a plan in place.

Chronic complications (Long-term consequences)

Over time, high blood glucose, high blood pressure, and high blood fat/cholesterol can damage your blood vessels. Blood vessel damage happens slowly. It may begin in childhood and continue throughout life. People with diabetes are more likely to develop blood vessel damage and get it at a younger age than those without diabetes. Often, you may not notice any signs of their presence until the damage has already been done. Regular contact with your healthcare provider is highly recommended.

The long-term consequences of diabetes can include:

1. The large blood vessels (also known as macrovascular or cardiovascular complications) lead to a heart attack, stroke, or circulation problems in the lower limbs and feet.
2. The small blood vessels (also known as microvascular complications) can lead to problems in the eyes, kidneys, and nerves, such as in the feet or other parts of the body, including skin, teeth, gut, and gums.
3. It can also affect sexual functioning.

Macrovascular (Large blood vessel) complications

In people with diabetes, atherosclerosis is the primary cause of damage to large blood vessels. Atherosclerosis occurs when plaque, which consists of cholesterol and other blood fats, accumulates inside the walls of blood vessels. Consequently, the blood vessels narrow, and the circulation of blood in the organs is reduced. Upon rupture of the plaque, blood clots can form, which can completely cut off the blood flow to the organs and other parts of the body. This can severely affect the blood vessels that supply blood to the heart, brain, and lower limbs.

Heart Health

A heart attack occurs when the blood supply to the heart muscle is interrupted. Blood is necessary to provide oxygen to the heart. Without blood, the heart cannot function. As a result, some of the heart muscles can be damaged or die down. The symptoms of a heart attack may include severe pain in the centre of the chest or a feeling of crushing. The pain or crushing sensation may move up the neck or down the left arm or may result in difficulty breathing. These symptoms are less common in women. Sometimes a person with diabetes may not have any symptoms of a heart attack as a result of nerve damage as it dampens the sensation of pain.

Brain Health

A stroke occurs when blood flow to the brain is blocked. Eventually, without blood, the brain can't get the oxygen it needs, and part of it gets damaged or dies. Similar to the heart, when the blood flow is cut off by a build-up of fat and cholesterol in the blood vessels, it leads to the brain (atherosclerosis). This type of stroke is called an ischemic stroke. It is the most common type. If the blood flow is blocked only for a brief time, it is called a transient ischemic attack (TIA). Your body may release enzymes that dissolve the clot quickly and restore blood flow. If you have TIA more often, your risk of ischemic stroke is high.

Another type of stroke is called a haemorrhagic stroke. It occurs when a blood vessel in the brain leaks or breaks. The most common cause of this is high blood pressure (hypertension), as high blood pressure weakens the blood vessels, which are more likely to leak or break.

According to a long-term study involving approximately 50,000 participants over a period of nineteen years, it has been found that a person with diabetes and hypertension has approximately a four-fold increased risk of stroke. You should contact the emergency room immediately if you notice any of the following symptoms:

- Facial drooping (drooping on one side of the face)
- Arm drooping (weakness or numbness down one side of the body)
- Difficulty in speaking

Lower Limbs

When the same phenomenon happens to blood flow to the lower limbs, it affects your legs and feet. This is called peripheral vascular disease. It can cause pain, cold, and a change of colour to the lower legs and feet. It can also cause slow healing of wounds, cause shiny skin on the legs, and pain in the buttocks, thighs, or calves while walking. The long-term lack of blood flow to the lower limbs can lead to ulceration and infection. This can increase the risk of amputation.

Microvascular (Small blood vessel) complications

Eye Health

People with diabetes are more likely to get an eye disease than people without diabetes. The three main eye diseases that people with diabetes get are retinopathy, macular oedema, cataracts, and glaucoma. Over time, the small blood vessels in the retina can become damaged and leak fluid or bleed. This is called retinopathy. Retinopathy is the most common problem and carries the highest risk of reducing your vision.

A cataract clouds the eye lens, blocking light from entering the eyes and causing poor vision. Glaucoma is a build-up of fluid in the eye, causing increased pressure. This pressure can damage your optic nerve.

Eye conditions can be managed more successfully if they are found and treated early. Have your eyes checked by an optometrist or ophthalmologist (eye specialist) regularly to look for early signs of damage. Early detection and treatment of eye problems can provide the best results.

Nerve Health

Nerve damage is called neuropathy. Neuropathy affects the nerves outside your brain and spinal cord. These are called the peripheral nerves. Damage can occur to the nerves in the legs, feet, arms, and hands. This is called peripheral neuropathy. Damage to nerves can cause pain, tingling, or numbness. There can also be damage to the nerves affecting your stomach (gastroparesis), intestines (diarrhoea or constipation), bladder (incontinence), or genitals (erectile dysfunction in men and sexual dysfunction in women). This is called autonomic neuropathy.

Kidney Health

Kidneys clean your blood. Your blood flows through filters in your kidneys. In healthy kidneys, the filters let waste pass out to your urine while retaining useful components in your blood. But having diabetes and hypertension causes high blood pressure. High blood glucose levels can damage the small blood vessels in the kidneys. This causes the tiny blood vessels that filter the blood to leak. As a result, the kidneys do not work as well as they should. This is called diabetic nephropathy or diabetic kidney disease.

Have your kidneys checked at least once every 12 months by your doctor. This will involve a urine test and a blood test as part of your annual diabetes check-up.

Other complications
Teeth and gums

There is a higher risk of dental problems when blood glucose levels have been above the target range for a long period of time. Dental problems can include tooth decay, gum infections (gingivitis), and gum disease.

Tooth and gum infections can increase your risk of heart disease. Signs of dental problems include a dry mouth and sore, swollen or bleeding gums. It is important to brush your teeth twice a day and floss every day to prevent dental problems. Regular visits to your dentist will also help maintain oral health. You should also tell your dentist that you have diabetes.

Skin

Skin problems can include very dry skin caused by damage to the small blood vessels and nerves. There is a higher risk of skin problems when blood glucose levels are above the target range. To avoid dry skin, you can protect your skin by avoiding irritants such as hot baths and showers, scented soap, and household cleaning products. Use moisturisers every day but not between your toes. Treat any cuts on your skin promptly to prevent infection. See your doctor if you identify any skin problems.

Research studies showing optimum diabetes control can prevent painful complications.

Now that you have a better understanding of the consequences of diabetes on the body, your best defence against these complications is maintaining your blood glucose, blood pressure, cholesterol, and body weight in the optimum target range. The closer you are to your target range, the more likely you are to prevent or delay these horrific and painful complications.

Landmark Clinical Trials in Diabetes

Landmark clinical trials are pivotal studies that can dramatically change the landscape of medicine. In the field of diabetes, the landmark clinical trials discussed below have led to major advances in the management of diabetes complications. There is enough evidence from these landmark studies indicating that diabetes complications could be controlled and prevented in people with type 1 and type 2 diabetes.

1. The Diabetes Control and Complications Trial

The Diabetes Control and Complications Trial (DCCT) was ten years long (1983-1993). It recruited 1,441 subjects between 13 and 39 years old with type 1 diabetes mellitus. All participants were relatively healthy except for diabetes and were free of severe diabetes-related complications. The participants with newly or recently diagnosed type 1 diabetes received either intensive glycaemic control (i.e., external insulin pump or three insulin injections daily) or standard glycaemic control (i.e., two insulin injections daily). The important finding of this study was that the individuals in the intensive glycaemic control group had far fewer complications, and the chances of developing an eye disease, kidney disease, or nerve disease were all reduced by at least half.

The participants in the DCCT trial continued to be followed up in the observational Epidemiology of Diabetes Interventions and Complications (EDIC) study. After decades of follow-up, it was observed that, despite the HbA1c levels converging in the two study arms, one year after the study concluded, the intensive glycaemic control group continued to have a significantly lower rate of microvascular complications. To summarise, there was a 63% reduced risk of diabetes-related retinopathy (eye disease) after five years, 54% reduced risk of kidney disease after five years, 60% reduced risk of neuropathy (nerve damage) after five years, and 30% reduced risk of cardiovascular events (including heart attack and stroke) after 20 years. The risk of complications increased with higher A1C values.[63, 64]

2. The United Kingdom Prospective Diabetes Study

The United Kingdom Prospective Diabetes Study (UKPDS) was a landmark trial that followed 5102 participants with newly diagnosed type 2 diabetes and ran for twenty years (1977 to 1997) in 23 clinical sites based in the UK. The participants in this trial were divided into an intensive therapy group (on medications) aimed at fasting blood glucose more than 106mg/dl or 6mmol/L (tight control) and the conventional therapy group (diet and exercise) with fasting blood glucose less than or equal to 15 mmol/l or 270mg/dl. The results showed a 25% reduction in eye disease, kidney disease, and possibly nerve disease, previously often regarded as inevitable, which could be reduced by improving blood glucose and/or blood pressure control.

People with high blood pressure were further divided into two groups. Both groups were treated with drugs to lower blood pressure. One group maintained an average blood pressure of 144/82 mm Hg (tight control) and the other group maintained an average blood pressure of 154/87 mm Hg. People who control their blood pressure are less likely to suffer strokes, heart failure, vision loss, complications of the eyes, kidneys, and nerves, as well as diabetes-related death.[65]

This underscores the need for patients to closely monitor and manage their blood glucose and blood pressure levels to mitigate the risk of further complications.

Further, when the intervention trial finished in 1997, all surviving UKPDS patients were entered into another ten-year, post-trial monitoring program that proceeded until 2007. Similar to the DCCT, differences in glycaemic control were lost one year after the study's conclusion. However, a 24% reduction in microvascular events, a 15% reduction in myocardial infarction, and a 13% reduction in death were observed in the intensive control arm even for ten years after the study ended.[66]

3. Steno-2 Trial

Steno-2 trial, 160 participants with type 2 diabetes and microalbuminuria (a marker for kidney function) were divided into intensive vs. conventional glycaemic control and were followed for a total of a mean of 13.3 years. Again, despite convergence in glycaemic control after the end of the study, participants in the intensive control arm had a lower risk of heart disease and death. Later, 21 years of follow-up showed a marked reduction in risk of microvascular complications and increased lifespan with 7.9 median years.[67]

What is the legacy effect?

It is common to assume that when you take medication to treat a medical condition, the effects will start immediately and last for some time. For instance, when you take a glucose-lowering medication, your blood sugar levels reduce within hours of ingestion and could last for a few days. These landmark studies have indicated, however, that there may be long-term benefits associated with previous periods of glucose control and harm associated with previous periods of hyperglycaemia, a phenomenon known as the "legacy effect" or "metabolic memory." [68]

The first compelling data for the legacy effect emerged from the long-term follow-up of the DCCT. Similar results were found in the type 2 diabetes population in the pivotal UKPDS and the Steno-2 trial. Despite the convergence in glycaemic control after the end of the study, participants in the intensive control arm had a lower risk of diabetes complications.

What do large-scale research studies say about lifestyle choices and the prevention of diabetes complications?

Over the past decades, researchers have taken great interest in understanding if lifestyle changes can slow down the complications of diabetes and, if so, what dietary and other lifestyle factors can help. It can be hard to make sense of these research studies. Here,

I hope to clarify them. The studies listed below are the most credible and authentic in different ethnic populations.

4. Look AHEAD (Action for Health in Diabetes) trial

The Look AHEAD trial was one of the major trials that evaluated the benefits of lifestyle intervention. The researchers wanted to know whether long-term weight loss would improve blood glucose and prevent heart disease in people with type 2 diabetes. Intense lifestyle interventions (≥ 7% weight loss with calorie restriction and ≥ 175 min/week of moderate activity) may not have a direct impact on heart health, but show improvements in lipids and blood pressure, sleep apnoea, renal disease, fitness, and depression. Needless to mention, blood glucose control was significantly good in the intervention group, and this effect was evident until eight years of continuous follow-up.[69]

5. The researchers found that the maintenance of weight loss is difficult to achieve in real-world settings and suggested that it is important to avoid prioritising weight loss as a primary goal of treatment instead of shifting attention to improving blood glucose levels and reducing diabetes-related complications.[70]

5. PREDIMED Study

The PREDIMED study was designed to assess the long-term effects of the Mediterranean diet on incident cardiovascular diseases in men and women at high cardiovascular risk in Spain between 2003 to 2011. The study recruited 7447 participants, where close to 50% of the participants had type 2 diabetes. Four-year follow-up showed that the Mediterranean diet decreased incident diabetes by 50% compared with the control diet after.

And also confirmed that it protects against heart disease. In brief, the results clearly show that a high-unsaturated fat dietary pattern is better for cardiovascular health than a lower-fat diet.[71]

Second, the Mediterranean diets were successful in older persons at high risk of cardiovascular diseases, most of whom were being treated with antidiabetic, hypolipidemic, and/or antihypertensive drugs (medication for blood glucose, blood lipids and blood pressure).[72]

Third, given the age of participants, the results tell us that it is never too late to change dietary habits to improve cardiovascular health.

Further, several research studies have demonstrated that improving dietary choices reduces cholesterol, LDL cholesterol, triglycerides, blood pressure, and glucose levels.[73] This decreases the risk of heart disease. Lifestyle choices may not alone prevent diabetes, but they can also prevent or delay complications associated with diabetes if you are already diagnosed with diabetes.

Is there a legacy effect of lifestyle changes?

Twenty and thirty years after the Da Qing prevention trial (Landmark diabetes prevention trial from China), the rates of health complications, including cardiovascular disease (CVD) and CVD deaths, were found to be lower in people who had been in intervention groups for diet, exercise, or both.[74] The Look AHEAD trial found that interventions for weight loss resulted in benefits for people with type 2 diabetes, including improved diabetes management with fewer drugs, lower risk for advanced chronic kidney disease, and lower risk for CVD with fewer drugs.[75] Experts have pointed out that legacy effects vary depending on the intervention effort and behaviours during follow-up studies.

Overall, these results suggest that the glycaemic legacy effect is a long-term benefit (or risk) granted to individuals with early diabetes. If this benefit is not taken advantage of, it could be muted over time as the health of blood vessels changes, and they develop complications from diabetes.[76]

Take Home Messages

1. A summary of the landmark trials that show that careful blood glucose management can lower the risk of long-term health complications in people with type 1 or type 2 diabetes.
2. Besides blood glucose, optimum control of blood cholesterol, blood pressure, and body weight is equally important for preventing and delaying the risk of diabetes complications.
3. People with diabetes need to gain control of their blood-sugar levels—fast. The years immediately after diagnosis (up to 10 years) are strikingly critical in terms of their future risk for heart attacks and death.
4. It is never too late to change lifestyle habits to avoid or delay complications of diabetes.

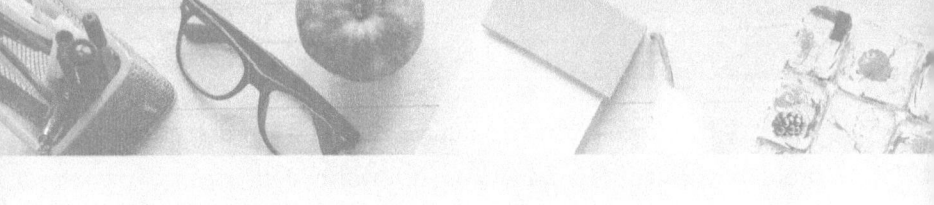

CHAPTER 5

INTRODUCING THE 5 C'S

THE 1ST C – CONDITION YOUR MIND

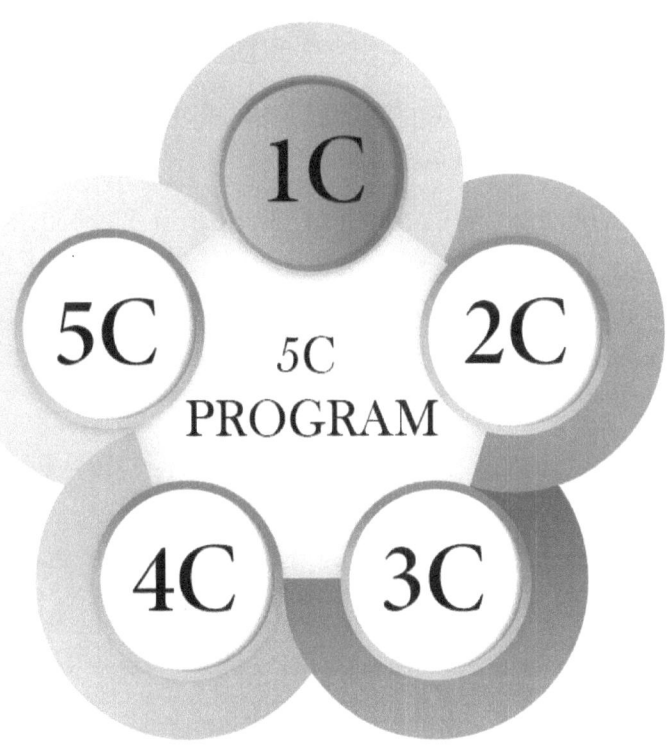

When you are told that you have diabetes, or that there is a problem with your blood glucose or insulin levels, or that you are "prediabetic" or borderline," there are often one of two reactions. Denial and anger or panic.

Once the doctors have told you about your situation, the denial phase can kick in. You might end up thinking, "Well, it's only PRE-diabetes, nothing to worry about," or "I've just been eating badly recently, it will be easy to put this right."

If you relate to this, it's OK. It's normal. And denial gives you some time to process and understand the situation. Anger is also a common reaction and it is often targeted at someone or something else. That's where the blame game starts, which can lead to the dangerous trap of feeling guilty or self-pity.

Either way, you are reacting to a stressful situation in a way any normal human would.

As described by Swiss-American psychiatrist Elisabeth Kübler-Ross in 1969, there are five stages of grief. These stages shift from denial, anger, bargaining, depression, and finally, acceptance, where one says, "It's going to be OK. I can deal with this. I may as well prepare for it."[77]

We also need to understand that grief is different for every person, and not everyone will experience all five stages. You may not go through them in this order, and there is no definite timeline.

Please, remember that it isn't helpful to judge yourself. Instead, prepare yourself to embrace the situation and acknowledge that you need to fix something which is not right. It is never too late to start a positive change in your life. The key is to be kind and patient with yourself because you are your best friend, philosopher, and guide in the journey of health and happiness.

Managing prediabetes and diabetes is about bringing change. You are in your present health situation partly due to your lifestyle up until today, so if you don't change the cause, you will get the same effect. It's like the saying "what goes around comes around." If you keep making the same choices, you will keep getting the same results.

For some, it could be just a few small changes, while for others, it could be a dramatic shift, and this is based on how far you are from your best lifestyle choices. The journey of change starts from your mind, moves to your body, and repeats until it becomes a subconscious habit or routine.

The first step in this journey is to condition your mind for the change.

What do I mean by conditioning?

Conditioning or preparing your mind is the first step to bringing any change in life. **It is a process of training your mind to become aware of and modify your thoughts, attitudes, thinking patterns, and beliefs to create a physical change in choices and behaviour.**

How do you condition yourselves for a change?

To understand the building blocks of conditioning, let me use a simple metaphor of a tabletop with sturdy four legs. If even one leg of the table is missing, it will not stand on its own. I call these four legs the four T's. Each is equally important for conditioning your mind for a sustainable lifestyle change.

The four T's of conditioning are:

1. Tune Your Motivation
2. Take A Decision
3. Track Your Belief System
4. Trace Your Emotions

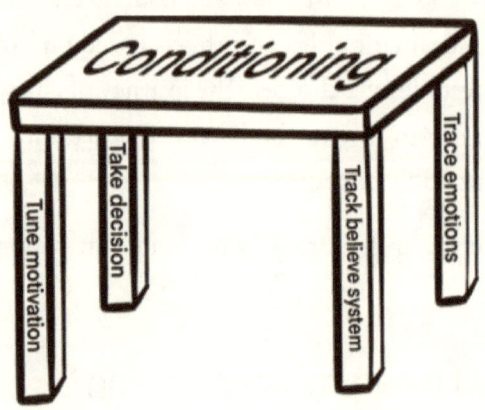

Tune Your Motivation

The simplest definition of motivation is, "wanting something desperately." What drives our determination to change is when we ask the right questions. The wrong question in this situation would be, "Why me? Why do I have to have this condition?" That is a victim mentality. The right question might be, "Why would I want to change my blood glucose, eating behaviour, weight, and blood pressure?"

Then, check your answer. If the answer is, "Because I want to live. I want to be healthy and be around for the people I love, and achieve my best life," that's good. If the answer is, "Because the doctor said I have to," then, check in with yourself again.

It is well known from research that lifestyle changes are much more likely to stick when they arise from within us rather than from external sources.[78, 79] In other words—it is something YOU want, something that is important to you.

For instance, imagine you have started a diet to lose weight to make your partner happy. In this case, you might lose weight, but you have painful memories of the process, and you feel you are forced by an external source to the cause of this induced pain, and your subconscious mind connects this pain to weight loss. In addition, these forced changes are not sustainable for a long time. What you have learned in this process is:

- Losing weight is a painful process
- Dieting causes me to lose weight, but when I stop, I gain more back
- Diets suck. I'm not doing this again

The emotions of disappointment, guilt, and failure are now associated with diet and weight loss.

Now, let's look at losing weight from the perspective of internal motivation. You ask yourself, "Why do I want to lose weight?" The answer is, "Because I want to feel healthy and be pain-free."

Approaching the challenge this way, you must decide not to judge yourself, or put unrealistic expectations on yourself. You are doing this for yourself, and it will take as long as it takes. The thought processes then become:

- I can achieve changes, and it gives me self-confidence.
- I can have good days and bad days but continue with the journey without fear of criticism or judgment. One bad day is just one bad day, tomorrow will be better.
- I feel happy with my progress.

When you lose weight, your subconscious mind feels a sense of achievement with pleasure and not pain. The emotions that follow are self-esteem, contentment, and satisfaction.

With any health challenge, you must look inside and find the internal motivation that is close to your heart, and work on your health because it is your best asset. You can start the journey at any stage, it is never too late.

Without conditioning your mind to think differently and finding this internal motivation, and a big enough reason why, old habits will come back as soon as things get tough. Hence the term "yo-yo" dieting, where someone tries to diet by following the "rules" of the diet alone, but without changing their fundamental beliefs about themselves and the reason they are 'dieting.' Will power only works long-term, when the mindset supports it.

Another error often made is to focus on the outcome and forget about the journey. What I mean by this is that people will think things like, "When I lose 10 kilograms, I will be happy." Feeling happy and proud of every achievement, whether big or small, is key to achieving the ultimate outcome. You can't wait to be happy. Be proud of yourself right now, for the choices you are making today.

Take a Decision

Take a moment to think about where you were 10 years ago. What were your health priorities then? What was your diet like and how did you deal with stress?

If someone asked you then, "Where do you see your health in ten years?" what would have been your answer? Are you where you wanted to be ten years ago? Whatever your answer, it is true that wherever you are today it's because of the decisions you have made.

Everything that happens in our life is a result of a decision. Not deciding is also a decision, right? If you have decided not to bother about what you eat, that is a powerful decision that will eventually affect your health outcomes.

You cannot turn back time, but if you accept that you are the master of your destiny, then you can alter your future. So, where do you see your health in the next ten years? How will you choose today to create the tomorrow that you want?

It is all about today, as rightly quoted by Albert Einstein: "Insanity is doing the same thing over and over and expecting different results."

Unless you decide to change your lifestyle choices, you keep fueling the flame of diabetes. You will only be treating the symptoms and ignoring the cause.

If making decisions is so simple and powerful, what is stopping you from taking them? Sometimes it can just seem too hard. You might feel that it's not your fault that you have diabetes or are pre-diabetic and now that you are, it is just too hard to do anything about it. Of course, it is true that genetics and other unavoidable factors such as age and ethnicity can play a role in developing diabetes. However, the good news is that there are steps you can take to manage it and even prevent it from getting worse. But it all starts with a DECISION.

You first have to know that is possible. Then it is important not to look at the whole journey but just the first step. Being smart about your decision will enable you to move forward without being overwhelmed.

Make sure your decisions/goals are specific (S), measurable (M), achievable (A), relevant (R), and timebound (T). Instead of deciding, "I am going to lose lots of weight quickly," choose, "I am going to make healthy food choices today, walk for half an hour and do half an hour of meditation."

If you are in a place of overwhelm it is OK just to look at today's choices. If you are feeling mentally strong, you can look at this week or this month. And that is all you need to do. You don't have to plan the next 3 years, that will feel restrictive and too big of a mountain to climb.

Decision-making demands clarity and achievability.

"Decide" is a mighty word that shapes our destiny. Everything that happens in our lives starts with the small and big decisions we choose to make. In today's world, it is easy to access the tools and resources required to acquire a positive lifestyle, but the most crucial challenge is the moment of decision-making.

This moment sets in motion your dreams into small steps which create your new reality. Stay committed to your decision, but bring flexibility into your approach, which we will discuss in later pages. The human desire to be healthy is eternal, but the path to reach that has building blocks of small and big decisions.

Now that we have decided to make small changes that would lead to more confident bigger decisions, let's embark on this journey. And, if you don't make any decision about your health and lifestyle, then you've already decided, haven't you?

Track Your Belief System

Eating is one of the first and most basic of human needs which starts from the day you are born. We keep eating several times a day, and it becomes a practice. But have you ever thought to yourself, "Why am I eating this?" The usual answer to this would be, "Because I like it," "Because I am hungry," or "It is what my parents ate." How you answer will tell you something about your belief system.

What do you mean by belief system?

Every experience of eating gives you a new learning or reinforces the beliefs you have acquired earlier. These beliefs come from experiences in the past. Why do you feel happy when you see a cake? Because you relate it to celebration or being 'treated' probably more than the taste or flavour of the cake.

Similarly, why do some people dislike soup or salads? It might be because we have had them when we are feeling sick or on a diet (depriving ourselves), and nothing to do with the actual taste of soups or salads. Our beliefs are often at such a strong level of certainty that we close or block ourselves to any new input or change.

There is an even stronger level of belief and it's called conviction. If your belief is associated with emotional intensity, where you hold it very close to your heart, it is called a conviction. A person with conviction will forever be reluctant to question his beliefs and might get defensive or annoyed to the point of argument or even obsession.

Of course, convictions are not always wrong. On the contrary, they have the power to drive action and overcome hurdles. However, when they are limiting you or preventing you from doing something that would benefit you then it might be time to re-evaluate.

For example, it is a Jehovah's Witness's conviction that 'you shall not sustain yourself with the blood of an animal' and therefore they refuse blood transfusions, even in life-threatening situations. To someone who is not of that faith, it can seem like a crazy decision. But they believe doing so would 'save the body but lose the soul.' Their conviction is strong—often frustrating the physicians trying to serve them. And it is clearly harmful to the body, but they believe it is necessary to save their soul. That belief is their right, and also their choice.

I also experience that type of conviction with patients who strongly believe that healthy food is distasteful, and they would prefer eating unhealthy and feeling happy, to eating a healthy distasteful meal. The definition of taste is very subjective and emotionally driven. It is very hard to change convictions, and you need an even bigger reason to do so.

So how do you change your beliefs? It is a simple process, but not always an easy one!

5 Steps to Create a New Belief

1. **Identify the (limiting) belief.**
   Example: I have to eat chocolates to feel good/I have to smoke when stressed/I have no time for exercise/I can't lose weight as diets make me hungry all the time.
   Ask yourself:
   - Do you strongly feel you are right?
   - Do you get disturbed or defensive if asked to change or challenged on the belief?

   If the answer is yes, acknowledge that you have a belief and that the belief is just that—a belief and not THE TRUTH. It is only the truth until you change it.

   Once you have identified the belief you need to unpick it. Let's take the example of – I can't lose weight as diets make me hungry all the time. Ask yourself the following: Is it true that I was hungry ALL the time? And if I was, was it really hunger or just a desire to eat (appetite)? A good way to test this is to allow yourself to eat something you don't really like anytime you feel hungry. If you really don't like apples, and you are genuinely hungry you will still eat it, but if it is only a desire to eat/craving/appetite, you will find it easy to refuse.

When you had this feeling of being very hungry all the time, were you on a very restricted diet? Were your weight loss goals realistic? Were you doing this diet because you wanted to or because you felt you 'should'? When you dig into the emotional connection behind the belief, you will unravel the truth.

2. **Start a new positive belief.**

   Example: There are other activities that make me feel good. I have time to exercise.

   There are other things that can make me happy when stressed. I can lose weight if I do it the right way for me.

3. **Strengthen your belief with facts and references.**

   Be a researcher, do your research from credible sources, read, talk to people who have done it or watch real-life stories. The more references you check, the more you connect emotionally. Example: Read books or watch YouTube videos about people like you who have lost weight. Research about calorie deficits. Focus on long term success stories rather than quick fixes. Talk to your doctor or health practitioner. Speak to people who have achieved what you want to achieve.

4. **Ask yourself:**

   What happens if I don't change the way things are?

   Meet, talk and share experiences of ill health as a consequence of obesity/diabetes. Watch documentaries or videos which highlight the consequences of lifestyle diseases like obesity, diabetes, and cancer.

5. **Reinforcement of the new belief.**

   The way to replace an old unhelpful belief with a new one is by repetition and reinforcement/reward. Whenever you do the new behaviour, acknowledge, appreciate, reward, and feel good about yourself. When you do this regularly, it becomes a regular behaviour and stays in your belief system.

Trace Your Emotions

Have a plan for feeling happy before you feel sad. What do I mean by this? We all feel low, angry, depressed, anxious, sad, and awful, sometimes. This is natural. Remember, whilst these emotions are natural, your eating choices can be profoundly affected by the way you feel. Big eating problems are often created because eating has become the primary source of venting emotions and achieving comfort or pleasure for a limited time.

This is not just about thoughts and feelings. There is a lot of neuroscience and physiological facts which make you feel this way. However, that doesn't mean there is nothing you can do about it. The most effective way to manage this is to start making a list of things that give you a similar feeling of comfort and pleasure. Note that this list should be at least between 15 to 20 activities, or else you will very soon run out of ideas for non-eating pleasures and replace emotional eating with one of these.

For instance, your list could include talking to friends, watching a film, listening to music, taking a bath, having a massage, reading a book or a magazine, playing with your children, family activities, shopping, finding a new hobby or skill, volunteering, socializing, walking, meditation, drawing, writing a letter or a journal, going to the spa, walking your dog, visiting a museum, dancing, singing, etc.

Remember, having a plan to make yourself happy when faced with a negative emotion will stop you from finding solace in food. Repeatedly practice these new activities when anxious, stressed or angry, and soon your subconscious mind will not seek food for comfort. So, have a plan for feeling happy before you feel sad.

Condition Your Mind for Mindful Eating:
Have you ever thought about why you eat what you eat?

This is a powerful question to ask yourself. In medical practice, we say that if you do not make the right diagnosis, how can you give the right treatment?

And Steve Jobs said, "If you define the problem correctly, you almost have the solution".

In recent years, neuroscientists have concluded that doing an activity a certain way, again and again, gradually creates neural pathways in the brain so that the behaviour becomes automatic (unconscious act), without any conscious effort. This process is called procedural learning.[80]

One of the classic examples of procedural learning is your eating behaviour.

Each culture has a certain eating pattern with no obvious rational explanation. It could be having coffee after meals, having a salad before meals, having dessert after dinner, or having popcorn with movies. You eat in a certain pattern because you have been doing this for years without any active thought. But on a neurological level, following such eating habits are simply habits and not necessities.

To make this simple, ask yourself before a meal, why do I eat what I eat? The answer to this question most often will be a packaged response-including series of micro-events all linked together. For instance, I chose to eat this because it is easy to prepare, I don't like to cook, I like the taste, it makes me feel happy, and so on.

Now pause and think about the real reason and whether it is the right choice. In other words, "pay attention." Simple as it sounds, it can be revolutionary and liberating. We call this being mindful about what, why, how, and when you eat.

The good news is that our brains are "soft-wired," not "hard-wired." They can be rewired with new neural pathways, which is called neuroplasticity.[81] Although this is not a quick and easy process, it takes intention, time and practice. Indeed, you have learned with time and practice, and remember it will take time and practice to "undo."

For example, it took years of repetitively having dessert after a meal or enjoying chips and soda with your favourite TV shows. You'll need some time to get used to switching to something less calorie-dense or stopping it altogether.

What is mindfulness?

Mindfulness is the basic human ability to be fully present, aware of where we are and what we're doing, and not overly reactive or overwhelmed by what's going on around us. Mindfulness is a quality that every human being already possesses. It's not something you have to learn in itself; you just have to learn how to access it.

This was translated into an 8-week Mindfulness-Based Stress Reduction (MBSR) program by Jon Kabat-Zinn back in 1979, and thereafter, this technique became a part of mental health practice.[82] Hundreds of hospitals and mental health centers now offer MBSR to help people with the relief of anxiety, stress, depression, chronic pain, and other conditions.

The dramatic success of MBSR in stress management and well-being has encouraged it to open its door to understanding the power of automatic and reactive behaviour called mindful eating.

What is Mindful Eating?

Mindful eating is paying attention to what you are eating and the reason for eating it, moment by moment, without judgment. It helps you focus on being present in the process of selecting, eating, and enjoying food. Slowly and gradually, being present shifts your eating habits. It helps with choosing and eating food in a certain way, teaches you how to taste your food, recognise your actual levels of hunger and fullness, and be accepting of your food preferences.

Mindful eating skills include paying closer attention to your body's hunger cues and learning to savour your food, which can help you change unhealthy eating patterns, control your blood glucose spikes, and lose weight. Recent research is repeatedly indicating that mindfulness and mindful eating is beneficial for weight reduction, calorie intake, blood glucose control and eating habits.[83]

Steps for Mindful Eating

1. **Be Here. Be Now.**

   Have you ever heard a parent say to their kids, 'Don't talk while you're eating'. As much as it might be so that they don't choke on their food or spray food particles on others it is also mindfulness! When you are mindful of what you are eating, not being distracted then you can fully enjoy it. In this way, you can also be aware of when you are becoming full.

   You might be thinking, "How does being present shift your eating habits?" First and foremost, it disassociates you from the feelings/emotions you are presently in. For instance, if you are feeling bored, stressed, anxious or angry, you are more likely to overeat or eat unhealthily to suppress your feelings rather than your real hunger.

   Secondly, it allows you to identify and be aware of the feeling of hunger and satiety (feeling full). Lastly, it gives you the opportunity to assess the taste of food more consciously and adapt to new tastes. Try this simple activity to bring your attention to the present. Raisin meditation.

What is Raisin Meditation?

Raisin meditation is a mindfulness exercise that requires you to focus your mind on the present moment using all of your senses— what you can see, hear, smell, taste, and touch. The idea is that by focusing all your attention on the tiny raisin (you could also use other food items, for example, date, fig, nut, dark chocolate), you help to bring your mind into the moment and train it to notice the present. Try for five minutes daily for at least a week. Evidence suggests that mindfulness increases the more you practice it.

How to do it?

Holding: First, take a raisin and hold it in the palm of your hand or between your finger and thumb.

Seeing: Take time to really focus on it; gaze at the raisin with care and full attention. Let your eyes roam over the fruit and pick out all the details: the color, areas of light and shade, any ridges or shine.

Touching: Turn the raisin over between your fingers, exploring its texture. Maybe do this with your eyes closed if that enhances your sense of touch.

Smelling: Hold the raisin beneath your nose. With each inhalation, take in any smell, aroma, or fragrance that may arise. As you do this, notice if this triggers your taste buds or makes your tummy grumble.

Tasting: Place it in your mouth, noticing how your hand instinctively knows where to go. Don't chew yet. Just spend some time concentrating on how the raisin feels on your tongue. Turn it over in your mouth and feel its texture on the roof of your mouth. Take one or two bites of the fruit without swallowing it yet. Fix your mind on the sensations just released into your mouth. How does it taste? How does this develop as the moment passes? How has the raisin changed? Do the smaller pieces of fruit feel different?

Swallowing: When you feel ready to swallow the raisin, see if you can first detect the intention to swallow as it comes up so that even this is experienced consciously before you actually swallow the raisin.

Following: Finally, see if you can feel what is left of the raisin moving down into your stomach, and sense how your body is feeling after you have completed this exercise.

Try this activity with your favourite food and with your least favourite and see the difference. You will have a different perspective by the end of the activity. This process helps you to stop and think over the unconscious behaviour of eating and learn the skill of enjoying your meals all over again. Keep repeating this exercise now and then to redefine your mindfulness while eating.

Have a Beginner's Mind

Eating behaviours start to evolve during the first years of life. As a child, you learn what, when, and how much to eat through direct experiences with food and by observing the eating behaviours of others. This is where you get judgmental toward food, you develop your likes and dislikes.

In mindful eating, we need to rewind and try a nonjudging attitude towards food. When you eat anything, the first thing you do is judge the food, whether it is good, bad, or bland. If you want to be mindful, keep aside the judgment for a while. Have a beginner's mind, blunt your previous generalisations, allow a new experience, and be open to whatever you mean in the here and now.

You could be wondering, "How do I do that?"

a. Be patient. It takes time to be aware moment by moment. Chew a few times, and swallow. You are slowing your process dramatically for the full experience, letting the experience unfold rather than racing through it.

b. Trust your own experience, and do not get carried away with others' opinions regarding likes and dislikes.
c. Accept whatever comes up in the moment, and do not try to resist or reference it to previous experience. It is what it is.
d. Let go of your previously held expectations and generalisations. For instance, "exercise makes me eat more" in my previous experience. Do not generalise. Try with a fresh mind and be mindful of your choices. Is it the exercise or the feeling of rewarding yourself that leads to overeating?

Recognise hunger and eat before you feel too hungry:

Do you eat your meals when you feel hungry or when it's mealtime, when you're feeling bored, feeling anxious, stressed, or socialising? Before you can answer this question, let me help you identify hunger.

What is Hunger?

Hunger is the body's need to eat. When you are hungry, your body sends you signals, like rumbling at first, and if you wait too long to eat, you may witness fatigue, lightheadedness, weakness, shakes, or irritability. Hunger cannot be controlled; it is instinctive. The feeling of hunger is caused by low blood sugar levels and hormone changes that prompt us to eat.

What is Appetite?

Appetite is the desire to eat. Appetite occurs as a coordinated effort between your brain and your stomach. When you feast your eyes on your favourite food in front of you or even sometimes in a picture or video, the desire to eat is initiated. Even the mere thought of food can elicit the same emotional response.

But unlike hunger, appetite can be ignored. And since appetite levels are greatly influenced by your brain, and it is a learned behaviour, you can even learn to control and change the level of your appetite.

Appetite itself is a good thing. It not only brings the emotion of food and pleasure but also lets you select from a variety of food to fulfill your nutritional needs. But it can be easy for a person to let their appetite take over their better judgment, leading to overeating and obesity. Remind yourself of the difference between appetite and hunger. It can help you keep a more balanced attitude toward food and eating.

What is Fullness or Satiety?

In addition to the feeling of hunger and appetite, there is another feeling called fullness or 'Satiety.' Fullness/Satiation refers to the process that occurs during a meal and leads to stopping eating. There is a delay between eating and feeling full, which is why if you eat very quickly you can become over full before you realise you have had enough to eat.

There are hormones released by the intestines which tell the brain you are getting full. However, eating slowly isn't always the answer as people who are obese, for example, may suffer from leptin resistance, meaning that they are less responsive to satiety or pleasure signals from this hormone.

However, the mind and body are intricately linked; our emotions affect not only our minds but also our body. For instance, when you are anxious, you might feel physical signals of increased stomach growling or burning of the abdomen. Separating emotions from physical signals that indicate hunger, fullness, or other physical needs is the most challenging part of mindful eating.

Awareness of your hunger and fullness patterns is one of the foundations of developing appropriate eating behaviour. A simple 7-point scale will help you identify your state of hunger and fullness with meals.[84] I find it a very simple and beneficial tool that I use with my patients to help them gauge these feelings and be mindful of them when they have their meals.

How does this work?

This is a two-way scale and can be used to score the feeling of hunger when starting the meal and the feeling of fullness 30 minutes after starting the meal. Score the scale at 1 ("Very Hungry") with a midpoint at 5 ("No particular feeling") through 10 ("Very Full").

For optimum eating, you should start eating at a 3 or 4. Because you're not at an uncomfortable level of hunger, and the blood sugar in the brain isn't too low, you can still make rational, intentional choices about food and **stop eating when you reach fullness between 6 to 7.** This information is empowering and will help you learn if you often override your hunger and fullness signals.

You might realise that when you are stressed because of your office work, you often avoid eating meals and end up very hungry in the late afternoon and then grab anything that is calorie-dense to satisfy the hunger without listening to the fullness signals. Keep listening to your body. It talks to you and always signals you for the right choices, provided you LISTEN.

The more practice you have listening to your body's signals, the easier it will be for you to be in sync with your body's needs, and sticking to positive eating habits will no longer be a battle but a way of life.

Remember the happiness quotient after a meal is not related to how much you have eaten but to how you feel after eating (e.g., happy, guilty, disgusted)

Table 5.1 Hunger-Fullness Scale

Hunger-Fullness Scale	
1	Starving (You're so hungry you'll eat anything. May feel starved, low energy, dizzy, headache, and gnawing stomach)
2	Very hungry (It's hard to think straight and concentrate)
3	Uncomfortably hungry (stomach growling with hunger pangs at intervals)
4	Just hungry (time to think about what to eat, but you feel you can wait)
5	Neutral (Feel neither hungry nor full)
6	Satisfied (You are nicely satisfied)
7	Pleasantly full (You are comfortably full but not overly full)
8	A little too full (You're stuffed and feel overly full / bloat)

9	Uncomfortably full (Super full; Clothes feel tight. If you eat more, you'll feel sick)
10	Painfully stuffed (Extreme fullness that causes pain or sick feeling)

Once you've learned how to identify the hunger-fullness body's signals, you can have fun discovering your pattern. Remember that these sensations may be very subtle or strong; start by making the best estimate, and I promise you will improve over time. This information will give you valuable information about your eating behaviour, which you might have never explored before.

Keep in mind to notice only the physical sensations and not the emotions (we will learn about emotions in the next section). Remember, the Hunger Fullness Scale is a tool, not a rule. For some people, it can be helpful in identifying unconscious eating or overeating, while for others, an early focus on hunger and fullness can feel like a diet. If that's you, consider focusing on honouring hunger first before thinking about fullness.

Exercise: Hunger Fullness Tracker Log

A simple three-day activity can tell you a lot about your eating behaviour.

1. Copy the below table in your notebook. Start with three days, and remember, do not change anything in your eating pattern. Just be your regular self.
2. Every time you sit to eat your meal or snack, just take a few moments to ask yourself, "How hungry or full do I feel on a scale of 1 to 10?" and record it in the log. Once you have

finished your meal, ask yourself again, "How hungry or full do I feel?" and record the score.
3. After three days, spend a little time scanning the data. Observe what is your average score before eating and after eating. Learn new insights about your eating behaviour.
4. There is no right and wrong. This exercise helps you to be more aware of your eating pattern and habits.

Table 5.2 Hunger-Fullness tracker for the Day (Sample menu)

Meal-Time	Before eating- Hunger score	What did I eat	After eating- Fullness score
Breakfast- 8.00 a.m.	3 (grumbling stomach)	Croissants (2) with coffee (1 cup)	7 (Pleasantly full)
Lunch- 1.00 p.m.	4 (thinking about food, snack hunger, energy levels slightly low, slight empty feeling to stomach but no pangs)	Rice (2 cups) with grilled fish (60g) with salad (1cup)	8 (too full, slightly distended roundness/ fullness to your stomach)

Dinner- 7.00 p.m.	5 (neither hungry nor full)	Pasta with white sauce (1 plate) and cola (1 cup)	9 (uncomfortably full, yes I kept eating long past fullness)
Bed Time- 10.00 p.m.	6 (satisfied)	Chocolate chip ice cream (2 cups)	5 (just neutral)

Please note that this is not a recommended sample menu, but rather an example one.

Scoring interpretations before and after eating:

Before eating:

1-2: You may be waiting too long to start eating, which could cause overeating.

If you have a habit of waiting until you're extremely hungry, you may tend to gulp down anything and everything in sight, and willpower will go out of the window. The problem is not poor willpower but low blood glucose and other stress hormones which induce hunger response pushing you to eat as much as possible. This pattern is clearly observed during fasting.

3-4: You are optimally hungry before meals.

To eat mindfully, you should be in this zone before meals, so that you are not emotionally driven to eat

5-6: You may be eating more because of appetite than hunger.

Sometimes, you eat because it is time to eat, irrespective of your hunger. This zone usually drives you to eat because of appetite and you end up overeating.

After eating:

6-7: you recognise fullness at the right time and stop eating.

8-10: You tend to wait too long to stop eating (overeat).

Watch out for emotional eating

Some of the most powerful culprits that prevent you from changing your behaviour are invisible. **Emotion-driven eating** is the most common reason for wrong dietary choices. Most of the time, when we are eating for our appetite (feel like eating) and not hunger (feel physiological hunger cramps), it is emotion driven. People eat out of anger, sadness, stress, boredom, fatigue, happiness, or sometimes loneliness. Everyone does this occasionally, and it is normal eating behaviour to cope with these emotions by distracting them from the pleasure of eating. However, the problem arises when this is too often or the only method of coping, comforting, or feeling good.

What can we do about this?

i. **Mapping your emotions**: The first thing we need to be mindful of is to identify your emotions through a simple exercise called mapping your emotions. In this exercise, you learn to identify your physical cues corresponding to the primary emotions of anger, sadness, fear, and joy. We all could respond differently to each of these emotions. For example, when you are angry, you can feel your heart racing, tightening of your shoulder and neck muscles, grinding teeth, frowning your eyebrows, or sometimes drying of your mouth. Experience each emotion and feel how your body responds to it. How are your muscles? Your abdomen? Your face? Butterflies in the belly? Your posture. Once you can identify them, start connecting the dots between your emotions and your eating behaviours. Keep a journal as in the sample chart below. Note down your emotion without judging to assess your invisible culprit.

Table 5.3 The Food Emotion Journal

Time	What emotion I felt before eating	What did I eat	Was I hungry	What emotion I felt after eating
Breakfast- 8.00 a.m.	Stressed about meeting in the day	Croissants (2) with coffee (1 cup)	No	Guilty
Lunch- 2.00 p.m.	Relief that the meeting was good	Chicken sandwich (1) with fruit juice (1 cup)	Yes	Content

Dinner- 7.00 p.m.	Frustrated that I have household chores to do	Pasta with white sauce (1 plate) and cola (1 cup)	Yes, but I kept eating long past fullness	Guilt and anger
Bed Time- 10.00 p.m.	Bored watching TV	Chocolate chip ice cream (2 cups)	No	Hopelessness

Continue to map your emotions with your food intake for 3-7 days to understand a pattern. Once you step back and look at the bigger picture, you will understand if you are emotionally driven to eating behaviour which is making it difficult to change your diet.

ii. Connect emotions to eating behaviour. Emotions affect your moment-to-moment decision-making and subconscious behaviour response. If you find that your decisions are emotionally driven, then you need to investigate why you're angry, anxious, lonely, scared or stressed. Think of several specific things you could do to rebalance your life or lower your stress. For example, if you are frustrated with household chores then ask for help. And if you are bored, talk to a friend or plan a get-together. Identify the cues that trigger these emotions. For example, waking up late increases the early morning anxiety of being late for work. Surround yourself with people who make you feel accepted and happy. Read self-help books and listen to podcasts or programs that help you structure your thoughts.

Evaluating your life doesn't mean avoiding every stressor or going to live off the grid in a forest somewhere. You need to find your own balance in the chaos of life.

When Khadeeja, a 30-year-old mother of three working as a teacher, came to my clinic, she had been trying to quit emotional eating late at night. She spent the whole day doing her chores and after her kids went to sleep, she finally had—what she called—"my time" which she used by indulging in chips and dessert while watching her favourite TV shows. She believed this would bring her the happiness she had missed the entire day due to her heavy commitments and responsibilities.

She was also convinced that this hour was so important that she could compromise her sleeping hours to 4-5 hours every night. However, at some point, she started feeling exhausted during the day, was unable to concentrate and felt low. Not surprisingly, she gained weight, reported irregular menstrual cycles, and her insulin levels climbed to dangerous levels. Although she was motivated and decided to make a change, she was unable to crack the puzzle of restrictive eating during the day and emotional eating at night.

During a long conversation, we discovered that the root cause of her problem was a lack of attention to herself and a belief that eating high-calorie food would make her happy. She began by going for a walk in the late afternoons while listening to her favourite book or music three times a week, meeting family and friends or calling friends once or twice a week. She put a limit on office work at home and joining a carpool instead of driving for one hour helped her find time to connect with friends on social media. She felt better and was enjoying the happiness of doing something good for herself.

Six months later, she was eating better, sleeping better and was happy with herself. The conditioning of her mind had allowed her to begin a focused lifestyle change in what she ate and how she looked after herself which allowed her to manage her insulin levels and weight.

Remember, regardless of your external environment which may be full of temptations and triggers, or challenging and hostile, the internal foundation you've built will always be there for you. It is important to be aware of your thoughts, feelings, emotions, belief systems, and behaviour. It is vital to be conscious of what and why you choose to follow the lifestyle habits you do and to evaluate them with a non-judgmental mindset.

Be aware that this is not a contest between the good you and the bad you. You are bound to fail sometimes, but don't get discouraged if you experience setbacks. Instead, rely on your knowledge and wisdom to catch up. Remember that compassion for yourself is the most powerful tool you have.

Take Home Messages

- You are in your present health situation partly due to your habitual lifestyle, so if you don't change the cause, you will get the same effect.
- Conditioning or preparing your mind is the first step for bringing any change in life. The journey of change starts from

your mind, moves to your body, and repeats until it becomes a subconscious habit or routine.
- The building blocks of conditioning are motivation, decision-making, beliefs, and emotions.
- Mindful eating is paying attention to what you are eating and the reason for eating it, moment by moment, without judgment.
- Hunger is the body's need to eat, and Appetite is the desire to eat. Awareness of your hunger and fullness patterns is one of the foundations of developing appropriate eating behaviour.

CHAPTER 6

THE 2ND C - CHOOSE, COOK, AND EAT REAL FOOD

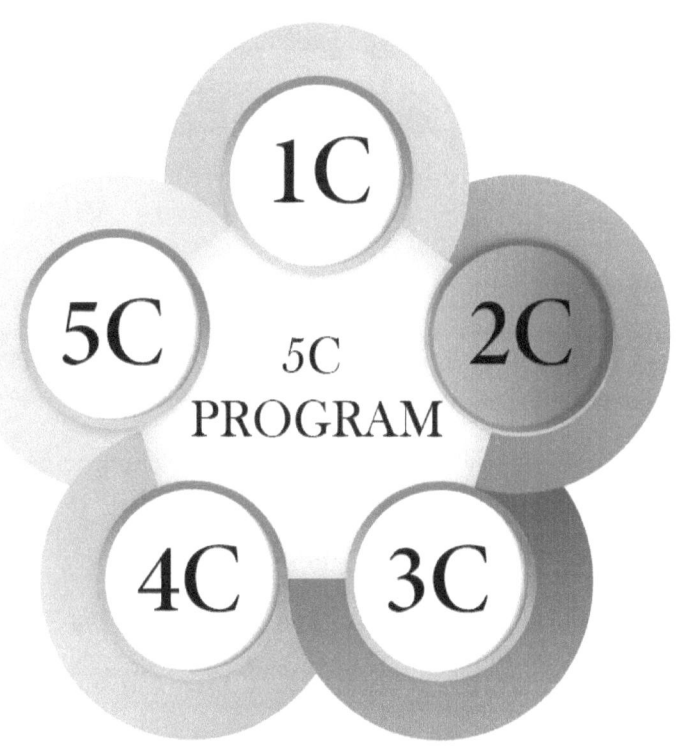

*T*ake just a moment and answer the following two questions. Your answers will be important to you as you begin to work on the 2nd C.

Question 1: What is real food?

Question 2: Why are you fond of the food that your mother or grandmother cooked for you?

We'll come back to the second question later. But first, let's talk about real food.

You don't need to be a scientist, a health expert, or a nutritionist to know what "real food" is and isn't. We, as humans, have the ability to identify what's good for us and what's not. Your gut instinct will kick in when you see an extra oily and greasy meal. It tells you that it isn't good for you, even if you feel the desire to eat it. Your mind knows the difference between real food and sham food. Let's take a look at two examples:

1. A glazed doughnut or soda? *Not real food*

2. A bowl of rice with stir-fried vegetables or a bowl of bean salad? *Real food*

Common sense may tell you that real food is clean, unprocessed, wholesome, and close to nature—the real organic produce that you pick from your garden or from a farm.

The next question is, "Do you choose real food"?

In today's world, where we are all hustling and surrounded by convenience foods stocked at our favourite supermarkets, which seem to make our lives easy and save us time, it is easy to forget that what we pick up for convenience is potentially damaging our health.

A healthy eating journey begins with making the right choices in the supermarket and understanding that the food items in your shopping cart have a significant impact on your health and therefore your quality of life.

The 2nd C is all about what food to choose and why, and how to prepare it.

Choosing Real Food

It's not always easy to choose the healthiest food. Things that look like they are good for you, might not be. In this section, you will learn how to identify real food by understanding how it's processed and handled on the journey to your dining table.

As little as a century ago, people consumed whole grains, legumes, fruits, and vegetables, as well as animal products, such as milk, eggs, and meat, in their natural, unprocessed state. To increase their shelf life and prevent spoilage, they would also process their produce minimally, such as drying and chilling fruits and vegetables, pickling vegetables, salting fish, and curing and smoking meat.

It was largely after WW2 that the food processing industry underwent enormous changes, including the mass production of canned foods, processed foods, cereals, sweets, and biscuits. In the 20th century, industrialisation laid the groundwork for modern food technology, which shifted the population's dietary habits. Further, as socioeconomic conditions across the globe improved in the second half of the 20th century, processed food products began to enter households either as foods that had a long shelf life such as canned foods or as foods that added new flavour and zing to everyday life like cookies and fizzy drinks, as well as processed meats and microwave meals.

Today our diets have become almost unrecognisable from those of our grandparents and great-grandparents. The way we shop, cook, and dine has altered our perception, attitude, and beliefs toward food.

As Wendell Berry (American Novelist and environmental activist) said, "People are fed by the food industry, which pays no attention to health and is treated by the health industry, which pays no attention to food". Hence, it's crucial that you understand the hidden secrets of food processing to protect your health from further damage.

Is Processed Food Good or Bad?

The answer is that food processing is not the issue. Food processing can be defined simply as any method used to turn fresh foods into food products. Human societies wouldn't have survived without food processing, as the benefit of food processing is increasing food availability. Most foods consumed today are processed in some way or another. Therefore, it's more important for us to understand the nature, purpose, extent, and effects of processing on our health and our well-being.

We need to identify the difference between the level of processing and nutrient depletion the food product has gone through.

As far as processed food products are concerned, they can range from minimally processed to heavily processed (also called "ultra-processed"). There are a few ways of classifying these food products, but it's somewhat arbitrary. The NOVA food classification system introduced by Carlos Monterio in 2017 is the one that's the most widely used in scientific literature. It groups all foods in accordance with the nature, extent, and purposes of industrial processing.[85, 86]

The NOVA classifies the food into four groups, which are based on the extent of their processing:

Group 1: Minimally Processed (or Unprocessed) Foods

Minimal processing is generally a physical process that's applied to a single food item. Its objective is to increase the food's preservation, accessibility, safety, or palatability. Examples of minimal processes include drying, chilling, freezing, pasteurisation, fermentation, fat reduction, and vacuum packaging. There is no addition of substances like sugar, salt, oils, or preservatives in these processes. Examples are frozen vegetables, pasteurised milk, and low-fat milk.

Group 2: Processed Culinary Ingredients

Food substances in this category are industrially extracted from natural sources or from group 1; for example, salt, sugar, honey, oil, butter, and flour. Essentially, these products are used as a seasoning for group 1 foods and are a part of home-cooked meals. Typically, you don't consume these products alone but rather use them to make meals by adding group 1 foods; for example, you don't consume salt, sugar, oil, and shortening alone, but you add them to flour to make bread, and you add salt and pepper to soups and broths. Example – plant or nut oils.

Group 3: Processed Foods

These products are made by the food industries by adding group 1 foods with group 2 ingredients to enhance their sensory qualities. They often are the revised version of the original food. Examples are bread, cheese, canned food, and smoked meat.

Group 4: Ultra-Processed Foods

The term ultra-processed food refers to an artificial food made from recombined ingredients and/or additives (group 2) or one that has been refined to the degree that it's no longer recognisable in its raw form. These food products are ready to eat or ready to heat with little or no preparation.

Their formulation is designed to reduce microbial degradation to give it a "long shelf life", to be transportable for long distances, to be highly palatable, and often to be habit-forming. For example, carbonated soft drinks, sweet or savoury packaged snacks, chocolate, sweets, and ready-to-heat prepared foods, such as pies, pasta, and pizza—these products are often referred to as "fast food" or "convenience foods."

The main aim of ultra-processed food is to make food convenient, tasty, and affordable.

Here's a simple litmus test for identifying ultra processed foods. Ask yourself:

a. "Can this food be prepared in the home kitchen?" If the answer is no, it's likely to be ultra-processed food.

And/Or

b. "Is it an industrial formulation with five or more ingredients?" If the answer is yes, then most likely, it's ultra-processed food.

For easier food selection, we will consider groups 1, 3, and 4 as the main groups and use the chart below as a guide board with examples. However, you should be aware that this isn't an exhaustive list and that some foods fit into multiple groups based on the level of processing. For example, bread can range from freshly baked with few ingredients to moderately processed whole grain bread to ultra-processed gluten-free, whole grain bread with artificial flavours and preservatives. I suggest that you always read labels to ensure that you are aware of the number and type of ingredients used in the product.

Table 6.1 Major Categories of Processed Food With Examples

Food	Unprocessed/ Minimally Processed Foods	Processed Foods	Ultra-Processed Foods
Grains	Whole grains, parboiled, or brown rice, whole grain flour, traditional bread, steel-cut oats, granola	pasta, noodles, instant oats, vermicelli	mass-produced packaged bread and buns, breakfast cereals, biscuits, cookies, cereal bars, pastries, cakes, cake mix, instant noodles
Fruits and Vegetables	fresh, chilled, frozen, vacuum-packed, 100% unsweetened fruit and vegetable juices	canned in syrup, brine, and oil; pickled vegetables	jam, jelly, sauces, ketchup, potato chips, mashed potato mix
Dairy	pasteurised milk, plain yoghurt, cottage cheese, fresh cream	milk powder	flavoured milk and yoghurt, ice cream, packed cheese

Meat	fresh meat, poultry and fish	salted, dried, cured, or smoked meats and fish; canned fish (with or without added preservatives)	sausages, nuggets, 'crab sticks'
Legumes	whole or split beans, lentils, chickpeas, red beans	soy protein	soy cheese
Nuts	roasted, unsalted	sugared nuts, nut butter (peanut, almond, hazelnut)	nut butter with chocolate
Fat		butter, margarine, ghee	
Beverages	tea, coffee, herb infusion	tea and coffee with added flavours	carbonated soft drinks, energy drinks, ready-to-make coffee and tea packs

Other			chocolate, sweets, (confectionery), chips, ready-to-eat meals, instant soups, frozen meals, preprepared ready-to-heat meals, burgers, pizza, meal replacement shakes and powders

*Note: We have not categorised group 2 separately but added to group 3 (processed foods) for easy comprehension.

Why is Ultra-Processed Food Unhealthy?

In the past four decades, the accessibility and intake of ultra-processed food products have increased in all countries, regardless of their economic level.[87] They have invaded our supermarket shelves, fast food outlets, street food outlets, kitchens, and refrigerators. It's a reality today that ultra-processed foods are here to stay. Epidemiological survey studies in big cities in many countries show that these foods constitute more than 50% of the daily calorific intake.[88]

These foods are convenient but come at a cost in terms of our health. Large population studies published in 2020 have reported the following evidence regarding their effects on health:

- Increasing daily intake of ultra-processed food increases the risk of type 2 diabetes (T2D). A population study on 100,000 adults showed that every 100gm add-on of ultra-processed food daily increased the risk of Type 2 diabetes by 5%. [89]
- A 9-year follow-up study of over 8000 Spanish adults reported an increased risk of overweight and obesity by 26% among participants consuming ultra-processed food more often. Processed meat, cookies, sugar-sweetened beverages and candies were among the major contibutors to ultra-processed foods. [90]
- Scientists found that the higher the intake of ultra-processed foods, the more likely to develop heart problems. Each additional weekly serving of ultra-processed food was associated, on average, with a 10% higher likelihood of cardiovascular disease within the decade. [91]
- Another interesting research from Spain on around 20,000 adults has shown that each additional serving of ultra-processed food could increase the risk of death by 18%. [92]

Does Ultra-Processing Change the Way Your Body Reacts to Food?

It's assumed that food is all about calories and macronutrients (carbohydrates, fats, proteins). Many of my patients ask whether two foods with the same calorie count can be substituted. I would answer both yes and no.

Your body's reaction to food is not only determined by nutrients it contains but also by the degree to which the food matrix is manipulated in processing.

Nutrition research has repeatedly reported that the impact of food is more than the sum of nutrients. It's also nutrient bioavailability (nutrients available for absorption), satiety (feeling full after eating), the hormonal secretions it triggers, and the fuel it provides to the gut microbiome, and more.

Think twice before switching from a 200-calorie wholesome sandwich to a 200 calorie cup of instant noodles. There is more to health than just calories; it is a whole package of wholesome nutrients that nature meticulously crafts.

How Is Ultra-Processed Food Linked to Diabetes?

Eating or drinking heavily processed foods — like sugary drinks, chicken nuggets, frozen dinners, or sweetened cereals — is associated with an increased risk for weight gain, heart disease, and even early death. A large observational study published by JAMA Internal Medicine in 2019 linked the consumption of such "ultra-processed" foods to high risk of diabetes.

Researchers evaluated the questionnaire responses of more than 100,000 diabetes-free people (average age about 43) over six years. People who ate the most ultra processed foods (about 22% of their diet) had a higher risk for developing diabetes compared with people who ate the least amount of ultra processed foods (about 11% of their diet).[93]

Why does ultra-processed food contribute to diabetes and poor glucose control?

Ultra-Processed Food Raises Blood Glucose Levels and Increases Insulin Resistance

Ultra-processed foods are generally unstructured, fractionated, and rich with free glucose and sucrose, which makes glucose easily available for absorption, causing a sharp increase in post-meal blood glucose.[94]

Various research studies have confirmed that the more processed a food is, the higher the glycemic index (glucose response) and the lower the sensation of satiety (fullness)[95]. This means that you would feel hungry more often, as a result of which you tend to eat more. Eventually, this cycle increases your blood glucose levels.

Refining grains enhance palatability (taste and flavour), lengthens the shelf life, and makes them easier to digest by removing fibre. Some examples of refined grain products are white bread, white flour, white rice, and degermed cornmeal.

Remember that fibre acts as a safety net holding the sugar molecules together. Therefore, removing fibre from the body speeds up the release of sugars and can indirectly promote insulin resistance by increasing body weight. Furthermore, dietary fibre also increases insulin sensitivity through fatty acids, thereby this protection is lost—a perfect recipe for type 2 diabetes.

Moreover, the food particle size also contributes to the glucose spike. The finer the particle size, the more surface area is exposed to digestive enzymes, the quicker the absorption of glucose, and the higher the glucose peak.

Do you ever wonder why you feel hungry an hour or two after you eat sugary breakfast cereal? These ultra-processed cereal products are made by destroying the natural matrix of the grains and loaded with sugar and additives to stimulate your brain's reward circuits.

But this comes at the expense of releasing more glucose into your blood, putting your heart, liver, and brain at risk. The millers split the cereal (wheat) into "white" refined flours, bran, and germ. This refined flour is used to make soft white bread or could be artificially reconstituted into several products.

Whole meal soft bread, for instance, is made from white flour mixed with a small amount of bran; whole meal wheat rusks contain wheat flour that has been blended with a long list of additives and ingredients, and the breakfast cereals that you love to eat as a quick breakfast are made from ground grain that is cooked and combined with sugar, starch, and a long list of additives for an amazing flavour.

This fractionation–recombination process makes cereal products that are high in energy levels, virtually devoid of protective fibres and micronutrients, of poor nutritional quality, poorly satiating, and hyperglycemic (high glycemic index). The manipulation of natural food structure isn't limited to grain but also extends to other naturally occurring foods like vegetables and fruits.

Several population studies highlight the protective role of whole grains (cereals) with respect to type 2 diabetes, heart disease, and certain cancers of the digestive tract. This role is attributed to fibres, minerals, vitamins, phytonutrients, and antioxidants. It's likely that the combination of several bioactive compounds in the right proportion and state is responsible for the complex protective effect of whole grains.[96]

Unfortunately, this complexity can't be created by supplementing these fragments of nutrients and phytochemicals in food, but we could create a new matrix with partial benefits.

In addition, the human body is designed to interact with these nutrients in a synergistic manner to produce a specific effect on health. The consumption of foods that contain added active nutrients (dietary fibre, antioxidants, phytochemicals, amino acids, fatty acids) appears magical, easy, infallible, and rapid; however, the consumption of whole foods appears realistic, time-consuming, complex, and requires effort. What's the reason?

The former focuses on partially correcting negative effects, while the latter addresses the root causes of negative effects over a longer period of time and doesn't exacerbate them. In short, it treats symptoms like hyperglycemia, constipation, or high blood pressure for a short period of time but fails to address the root cause.

Ultra-Processed Food and Feeling of Hunger or Craving for Food

In an experiment, scientists evaluated the feeling of fullness after eating a whole carrot (fibre and structure) vs. blended carrots (fibre but no structure) vs. carrot nutrients (prepared in the laboratory; no fibre or structure). Its authors reported that the feeling of fullness after eating whole carrots was the highest, concluding that the natural matrix structure of fruits or vegetables has a profound effect on how full you feel after eating.[97] A further example, is that eating a whole fresh fruit is more filling than drinking its juice.

Ultra-processed foods are a lot easier to chew, leaving a short time for the complete stimulation of satiety hormones. And they contain less protein and fibre than minimally processed foods and raw foods, with fibre and protein being the most satiating nutrients. Ultra-processed foods put your body in a chronically hungry, metabolically damaged, fat-storing mode.

In a nutshell, ultra-processed products are less satiating (i.e., an individual feels less full after eating) and more hyperglycemic (releases more glucose in the blood) than minimally processed or normally processed products.

Ultra-Processed Food and Gut Health

Our gut microbiome can be viewed as a bustling, overcrowded metropolis where people from diverse backgrounds live and work, contributing to the city's peace and well-being in their own way. This microscopic 'city' has trillions of microorganisms (also called microbiota or microbes) belonging to thousands of species of bacteria, fungi, yeast, and virus peacefully coexisting. In short, a microbiome is a community of microorganisms living together in a particular habitat. Us!

The intestines contain both helpful and potentially harmful microorganisms. In a healthy body, these two microbiomes coexist without problems. But if there's a disturbance in that balance, dysbiosis occurs, and this is the primary source of inflammation (the body's immune reaction to the irritant/insult) in the gut and throughout the body. As a result, the body may become more susceptible to disease.

Every person has an entirely unique network of microbiota that's originally determined by one's DNA and later influenced by the environment, medication use, lifestyle choices, and dietary choices. The interesting fact is that when you change the environmental exposures and diet, you can alter the balance toward good health or disease.

Ultra-processed foods that are high in refined carbohydrates, fat, and chemical additives (e.g., cookies, fries, desserts, sugar-sweetened beverages, and fast food) alter the balance of the microbiome causing dysbiosis and inflammation. Hence, making the foundation strong for insulin resistance, which is the trigger for the onset of type 2 diabetes.

These foods are deficient in nutrients that improve microbiome and gut health; for example, dietary fibre, polyphenols, and antioxidants that come from natural fruits, vegetables, grains, beans, and fermented products.

This potential gut disaster could be exacerbated further by an overload of sugar or simple carbohydrates (which are, of course, both also common in ultra-processed foods). Although, the potential pathways of how sugar intake might affect the gut microbiota aren't clear since sugars theoretically don't reach the colon as their absorption takes place in the small intestine. Some studies have shown that if we exceed the sugar-uptake potential of our small intestines, what's left over can also create a harmful breeding ground for microbes.[98]

In addition, there's also good evidence that consumption of a large amount of fructose within a short period of time (i.e. how candy and sugar-sweetened beverages typically are consumed) and even more so when fructose is unbound (as in products sweetened with high-fructose corn syrup) causes dysbiosis. Hence, an increased amount of fructose reaches the colon, which is suggested to contribute to a gut microbiota composition that associates with obesity and other metabolic diseases like diabetes, cardiovascular diseases, and certain cancers.[99, 100]

There's a laundry list of ways ultra-processed foods could mess with gut microbes—from certain food additives like emulsifiers to fat content to lack of dietary fibre. If any of these hypotheses turn out to be unsupported after further research, there can be a dozen more possibilities waiting in the ranks.

A simple example of our everyday meals will help us to grasp these tricky concepts.

Why is rice with stir fried vegetables different from instant rice noodles with vegetable flavour to the gut?

The main ingredients for boiled rice with stir-fried vegetables are minimally processed rice grains with cut vegetables fried in oil and spices. Here, their original plant cells are structurally intact.

But what if you ground the rice into fine flour and made rice noodles (added preservatives) and topped it with sauce constructed with natural vegetable flavour? Now there are no whole cells left, only the acellular compounds that were once in the foods. This makes the nutrients in the dish, in a way, already partly digested.

For bacteria living in the digestive tract, this means nutrients are available for them to eat sooner and in greater quantities since they don't have to break down any cell walls or membranes. A constant influx of quick-to-absorb nutrients could trigger an increase in the bacteria's growth, an expansion of their territory, a change in their composition, or a change in their behaviour (i.e. what they eat or what by-products they produce).

Inflammation and Ultra-Processed Food

Inflammation is part of the body's defense mechanism. It's the process through which the immune system recognises and removes harmful and foreign stimuli and begins the healing process. Inflammation can be either acute or chronic.

As the name implies, acute inflammation comes rapidly, needs short-term care, and gets better when treated, such as redness, warmth, swelling, flu, pain around tissues and joints, or when you cut yourself. For healing, your body sends inflammatory cells to the injury. These cells, upon reception of sensations, start the healing process. In this way, inflammation is good because it protects the body.

In contrast, when inflammation gets too high and lingers for a long time, the immune system continues to pump out inflammatory cells and chemical messengers to heal. In other words, your body is under consistent attack, so the immune system keeps fighting indefinitely. When this happens, inflammatory white blood cells may end up attacking nearby healthy tissues and organs.

Research has repeatedly proven that chronic inflammation can turn into a silent killer as it's strongly linked to diseases like type 2 diabetes, heart disease, arthritis, and cancers, to name a few.[101]

Unfortunately, the problem is that chronic inflammation is often "invisible" since it doesn't show tell-tale physical signs the way acute inflammation does. So how do we know if we have high inflammation? A simple blood test measures a protein produced by the liver, which is known as the C-reactive protein (CRP). It increases in response to inflammation. A CRP level less than 0.9 milligrams per deciliter (mg/dL) is considered normal. Whereas,

between 1 and 3 mg/dL often signals a low, yet chronic level of inflammation.

The solution to reducing chronic inflammation doesn't come from the pills in the pharmacy, but from what you pick at the grocery store to cook in your kitchen. Ultra-processed foods are related to greater energy density, saturated and trans-fat content, added sugar, lower fibre, and micronutrient content—all of which are attributes of pro-inflammatory diets.

For example, foods like white bread, pastries, French fries, sugar-sweetened beverages, soda, steak, and hotdogs increase inflammation. A review of 53 research studies has reported a 37% increase in the risk of type 2 diabetes with a daily consumption of 50 grams of processed meat (preserved by smoking or salting, curing, or adding chemical preservatives; for example, sausages, bacon, and deli meat).

Alarmingly, the review also suggests that every two slices of bacon eaten daily nearly doubles your risk of developing type 2 diabetes. What about the most common ultra-processed food—sugar-sweetened beverages?[102]

Ultra-Processed Food Taste Mystery That Pushes You to Indulge in Overeating

Research of the science of flavours and the feeling of fullness (satiety) has shown that you have a certain affinity to each taste (sweet, sour, savoury, bitter), and you also have cravings for these distinct tastes. Moreover, we reach satisfaction more quickly when we eat one flavour rather than when complex flavours are involved.[103]

For example, a regular can of cola contains about 40 gm of sugar (8 tsp sugar). Even though you don't find it very sweet as it's wrapped with other flavours, it would be very unfulfilling, even awful, to drink a glass of water with 8 tsp of sugar, as this would be overly sugary and sweet in taste.

What happens is that the flavours play in your mouth. Your taste buds might start to sweeten but then be hit by a tangy cola flavour, then you feel the sweetness in your mouth, and revert to the tanginess, and so on. This experience is appetising but also delays the feeling of satisfaction.

Ultra-processed food companies are well versed in this science and use it to their advantage by playing with flavours and textures to create novel flavours, which make us eat more and more to reach the satisfaction level. In other words, reaching out to chips, crisps, candy bars, colas, or cookies is not a lack of willpower alone—you have a whole lot of science working against you.

We Live in a Time When Ultra-Processed Food Is All around Us—What Should You Choose?

So, how do we break our dependence on ultra-processed foods? You can start by learning which foods in your diet count as ultra-processed. You don't necessarily have to give them up. But once you know how to spot an ultra-processed food, it's easy to find a less-processed substitute.

In my opinion, the most effective way to resolve this issue is to develop a food-choosing algorithm—a mental program that runs in your subconscious mind when you are picking out food or deciding on a meal. This will help you to make a powerful decision that will improve your **health.**

Follow the four steps in this process:

1. Record everything you eat for three to seven days (including the weekend).
2. Identify how many servings of ultra-processed foods you consume daily by answering the two questions discussed earlier. First, can this food be prepared in the home kitchen? If the answer is no, it's likely to be ultra-processed food. Second, is it an industrial formulation that contains five or more ingredients? If the answer is yes, then most likely, it's ultra-processed food.
3. Make the switch to healthier whole foods and limit your consumption of these foods to one or two times per day.

Table 6.2 Examples of Switching Options

Ultra-Processed Food	Wholesome Option
White bread	homemade whole wheat or other grain bread; traditional homemade bread
Cola beverages/Soda	sparkling water/carbonated water with lemon and mint or a splash of real fruit juice or fruit slices
Sweetened breakfast cereals	oatmeal made with rolled oats and sweetened with fresh fruit
Fried chicken or Fish with fries	roasted or baked chicken or grilled fish with homemade sauce and vegetables
Flavoured yoghurt or milk	yoghurt/milk blended with fresh fruits

Food is more than fuel and filler—it's a relationship. So, the next time you head to the grocery store, remember to identify the ultra-processed foods and their ingredients. Read labels and add food to your shopping cart that has ingredient lists of things you recognise. Limit items that are high in added sugar and sodium.

Look for switching options and pick ingredients to prepare a meal at home with a focus on consuming more whole grains, beans, milk, yoghurt, fruits and vegetables (fresh or frozen), or canned nuts.

Let's look back at the question that was asked at the beginning of this chapter. "Why are you fond of the food that your mother or grandmother cooked for you?". The answer is of course, that it is made with love and associated with being cared for. Christy Fergusson, a British Food Psychologist conducted a survey in which 58% said they enjoyed food more if it was prepared with love and care.[104]

I would say it's more than that. It's a combination of natural ingredients, traditional recipes, and tailoring them to your family's tastes and preferences. Cooking the way Grandma did is an easy way to make your food healthier and less processed. The reason for this is simple—traditional recipes were developed before ultra-processed foods existed. Furthermore, they are tasty, we recognise their flavour, taste, and texture, and we serve them as our family food. As a result, these recipes are easy to adapt using fresh, natural ingredients from your own kitchen.

Cook Real Food

When you start to make these lifestyle changes, you will inevitably fail a few times at the beginning. It is bound to happen, like any other change in life. So, what do you do? Instead of blaming the lack of willpower for failure, look for the underlying causes. Often, the reason is inadequate planning.

The famous basketball coach, John Wooden sums it up saying, "Failing to prepare is preparing to fail."

One of the most important preparations before changing your food habits is learning the basic skills of meal preparation. Cooking your meals is a lot easier than you think, it's more fun and cheaper than eating out. Regardless of your ability, anyone can learn to cook. I recommend spending some time learning about planning, preparing, portioning, and storing your meals before you decide to change your eating habits. These tools are essential for a successful change in your meal plan.

In today's world, you see a revival of interest in hobby cooking inspired by the plethora of cooking programs on TV and on social media platforms. This has driven the demand for trying an array of exotic ingredients, and cooking methods. There has never been a better time than the current digital era, to find the knowledge and the tools you need.

The present global trend indicates that we have shifted from the "conventional sitting at the dining table eating home-cooked food with family" to the "eat as you go" model. This shift could be attributed to factors, such as busy lifestyles, more unconventional working hours, a rise in single households, and an increase in the number of working women.

A global survey in 2011 revealed that as many as 55% of respondents worldwide cook a meal entirely from raw ingredients on a regular basis (i.e. at least once a week), while 38% do so using some pre-prepared ingredients.[105]

Recent scientific literature suggested a potential link between increased home cooking and healthier dietary patterns[106]. Besides being healthier, preparing healthy food at home is more enjoyable. You can prepare tasty, nutritious food that meets your taste and fits within your budget. Therefore, choosing whole food ingredients and preparing them with love will go a long way in preventing and managing type 2 diabetes.

Ultra-processed food increases our risk of obesity, type 2 diabetes, cardiovascular disease, and cancer. Home cooking enhances our health as it incorporates more classic culinary ingredients, such as oils, sugar, ghee, butter, salt, and spices; it uses more classic cooking methods, such as steaming, braising, frying, or water cooking; it includes more classic mechanical treatments, such as grinding, sectioning, and peeling; and it uses classic fermentations, such as alcohol fermentation and lactic acid fermentation.

According to a study on more than 9,000 adults by John Hopkins in 2014, the results showed that people who frequently cook dinner at home consume about 150 fewer calories per day than those who cook less.[107]

Another research review of 41 studies reports that people who live alone—who are less likely to cook on a regular basis—often have diets that lack core food groups, such as fruits, vegetables, and fish, and a higher likelihood of having an unhealthy dietary pattern.[108]

A long-term study followed 58,051 women and 41,676 men for 26 years (from 1986 to 2012) and found that people who ate 11-14 meals every week at home had 14% less risk of developing type 2 diabetes than those who ate only six or less home-cooked meals every week.[109]

You could say that having 1-2 meals every week that are not home-cooked (e.g., at a restaurant, precooked) doesn't affect your risk significantly (although this is an estimation).

There are several research studies on people with type 2 diabetes that clearly shows home cooking interventions improve blood pressure, blood glucose, and weight reduction.[110]

Culinary medicine is an emerging field that aims to change the nutritional health of people by focusing on skills, such as food shopping, storage, and meal preparation. This emerging field makes it evident that the more you consume home-cooked meals, the healthier you live. There are several reasons for this, including the use of healthier ingredients (fewer chemical additives), healthier skills (less sugar/salt/fat and traditional cooking skills), and healthier eating habits (meal timing and family time).

Are you excited about the prospects of cooking more, or feeling overwhelmed and wondering where you can fit the time in? If it's the latter, remember what we discussed about behavioural change and refer back to Chapter 5. No matter your ability or experience, you can always start to improve your skills and reap the benefits. Several research studies indicated that a lack of cooking skills could also contribute to the reduced diversity of food eaten, leading to unhealthy choices.[111]

Table 6.3 Common Barriers and Empowerment

Barrier	Empowerment
I have no time or energy to cook.	There's always time for new habits. Remember, nothing comes above your health. Keep that as your motivator. Get help and offer help to make a meal together (e.g., a family member, roommate, friend, colleague). Pre-preparing and freezing basic items; for example, whole meal bread, sauces, using frozen vegetables/fruits, precook half meals, and freeze/store. Use kitchen gadgets like a chopper, blender, grill, pressure cooker, and many more to make preparation easier.
It's overwhelming. I don't know how to cook.	Start with small steps and easy recipes; for example, sandwiches, salads, wraps, boiling eggs or vegetables or rice. Make a practice of planning your meals a day ahead. Get help from family/friends. Use shortcuts; for example, buying pre-chopped or frozen vegetables.
It's tiresome and boring.	Play fun music. Listen to a podcast. Call a friend. Cook with a partner/friend/sibling. Make cooking time screen time.

Three simple steps to adapt to healthy meal preparation:

1. **Preparation:**

- Start with a few home-cooked meals every week (depending on your present count) and push to a target over time of up to 5-6 days a week.
- Give your kitchen a makeover by adding gadgets to make cooking simple and easy. You could start with a sharp knife, a simple blender, a vegetable cutter, or an air fryer. Don't forget to add measuring spoons and a food-weighing scale to help you measure your cooked portions before you eat.
- Ask your family/friend to help you to make the process fun and learning.
- Store semi-processed/pre-cooked food in glass containers in the fridge.
- Get a list of healthy ingredients that are natural and fresh (fruits, vegetables, whole grains, beans, nuts) and add a list of spices and go-to ingredients, such as vinegar, lime, homemade vegetable/chicken broth, fresh spices, ginger, garlic, mustard, and chili sauce.

2. **Get going:**

- Get inspired by healthy cookbooks, cooking shows, vlogs and blogs, and try new recipes. Prepare your go-to list with at least five main courses, four salads, three snacks, two sandwiches, and one dessert. Remember to be ready with these recipes before you start any dietary program.
- Start a new love affair with salad. No, not the lame two-ingredient kind you may have grown up with. An amazing, colourful, hearty salad can stand on its own as a main course.

- Push your cooking skill set by adding new cooking methods and techniques one at a time, like baking, grilling, and freezing. Check out social media and YouTube for support.
- Try making your own recipe journal. As soon as you are hands-on with a specific recipe and you are satisfied with the way it turns out, jot it down. You are on your way to your very own personal recipe cookbook.

3. **Storing:**

- Make extra portions to store. Making double portions of specific recipes, then freezing extra portions that can be conveniently reheated at mealtimes, saves time on working days. This is particularly handy when you are tired and not motivated to cook.
- Precook basic sauces/gravies. Prepare common sauces, chutneys, and gravies and portion them. They can be stored in the fridge or frozen. Use them as and when needed.
- Ready-to-cook ingredients. Prepping the ingredients required for specific meals ahead of time is a way to cut down on cooking time in the kitchen. For example, cut vegetables, blanch vegetables, freeze whole grain bread, and pre-make a batch of cooked rice or beans.

You can meal prep in many ways, depending on your goals, schedule, and preferences. Talk to your friends and colleagues, explore well-known websites, social media handles, YouTube, and much more.

Ultra-processed foods are designed to entice you and increase hunger cravings. They lead to health problems and chronic diseases.

Using the 2nd C, you can use homemade food to lower the risk of type 2 diabetes and other health problems. You are in control and you get to choose what does into your food. Chemicals OUT, nutrients IN!

Take home messages

- A quick test for identifying ultra-processed foods. Ask these two questions: "Can this food be prepared in the home kitchen?" If not, it's ultra-processed food; and "Is it an industrial formulation with five or more ingredients?" It's most likely ultra-processed if it's yes.
- A growing body of research indicates that consuming ultra-processed foods increases the risk of developing type 2 diabetes, cardiovascular disease and other health problems
- Consider switching to healthier whole foods and limiting your consumption of ultra-processed foods to one or two times a day.
- Research suggests that having 1-2 meals per week from outside sources is unlikely to significantly impact your health. However, as the frequency of outside meals increases beyond this threshold, the potential effects on health become more noticeable.
- A simple technique for healthy eating is to cook more at home rather than eating out. The key to preventing and managing type 2 diabetes is choosing whole food ingredients and preparing them with love.

CHAPTER 7

THE 3ᴿᴰ C - CREATE YOUR OWN MEAL PLAN

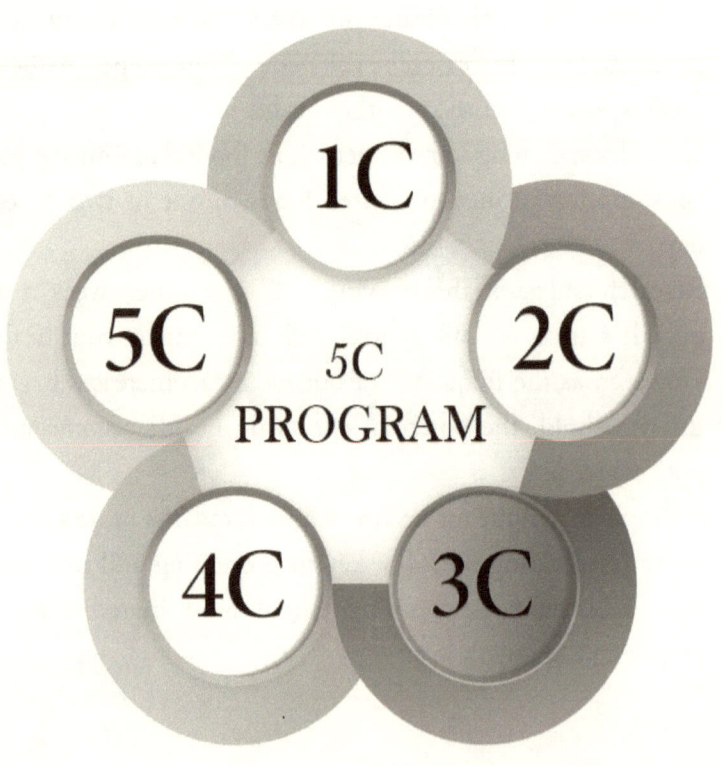

As the Supreme Commander during World War II and later the US President, Dwight D. Eisenhower said, "Plans are worthless, but planning is everything." It's not the plan itself, but the act of planning that lets you choose the best way forward on an unfamiliar path.

The 3rd C will prepare you to embrace the power of planning and unlock your full potential to turn your aspiration into reality. Even though planning may feel tough at times, it is a valuable investment in our future. Meal planning is no different! It may seem daunting and confusing at first, but by now, you are familiar with food groups, real food, macronutrients and their effects on blood glucose. We need to put the pieces of the puzzle together.

You might think, "Why can't I just get a meal plan with what to eat at each meal, and someone could cook it for me?"

Well, you can find people who will give you a meal plan, however it's not a great long-term option. Meal plans are often inflexible, leaving little room for adjustments or personalization. As a result, it can be challenging to stick to a rigid plan for an extended period. Moreover, relying solely on meal plans may hinder your ability to learn and develop a better understanding of nutrition.

By simply following a plan without actively participating in the decision-making process, you miss out on the opportunity to make informed choices. In the long run, building sustainable and healthy eating habits requires more than just a rigid meal plan. It involves learning about proper nutrition, experimenting with different foods, and discovering what works best for your unique needs and goals.

Remember, it's not about finding a quick fix but developing a sustainable and enjoyable relationship with food that empowers you to make better decisions for your overall well-being.,

Life is full of unexpected surprises and changes in your daily routines. This is especially true when it comes to sticking to a strict diet. We've all been there—everything seems fine until something happens that disrupts our plans.

It could be a work deadline that requires you to stay late at the office or a sudden conference that takes you away from your usual routine. In these moments, we often find ourselves drifting away from our meal plans. Why does this happen? It's because you haven't learned how to adapt healthy eating habits to your own tastes, preferences, and daily activities.

When you possess the skills to make responsible choices, you become the master of your own lifestyle. You have the freedom to enjoy occasional indulgences without guilt, as you know how to balance them with healthier choices. This flexibility allows you to maintain a sustainable and enjoyable approach to your diet and overall wellness.

You learnt how diet plays a significant role in blood glucose levels in chapter 3. Diet is the key to mastering diabetes.[112] By planning your meals to optimise your glucose levels, you will have room to make mistakes and you will be able to bounce back.

In Chapter 3, you discovered the powerful impact that diet has on blood glucose levels. It's clear that diet holds the key to mastering diabetes. By carefully planning your meals to optimize your glucose levels, you create a foundation that allows for flexibility and the occasional slip-up too.

It's important to remember that each person's body responds uniquely to changes in their eating patterns. Even individuals with the same weight, age, and duration of diabetes may experience different outcomes.

There's no rush, no stress, and no need to set unrealistic goals. Simply take your time, enjoy the journey, and listen to your body.

To kickstart your meal planning journey and make it enjoyable and effortless, I have laid out a comprehensive blueprint spanning four weeks. Each week is designed with three key components, outlined in the chart below. This structured approach will provide you with a clear roadmap to follow, ensuring a smooth and successful experience.

The first week of this program is crucial as it serves as a foundation for assessing your current state and establishing a starting point from which you can measure your progress over time. It provides an opportunity to set realistic goals, define benchmarks, and track your advancement towards them.

During this initial week, it is important to engage in honest introspection and self-reflection regarding various aspects of your lifestyle, including your dietary choices, daily activity level, sleep patterns, stress levels, and fluctuations in blood glucose. Take the time to evaluate who you are, recognizing both your strengths and weaknesses. This self-awareness will serve as a guide for identifying areas that require improvement.

In the second week of this program, we will delve into the art of understanding and selecting foods based on their nutritional value, and explore the concept of food groups. One of the key skills we will focus on this week is the ability to "fix your plate" by creating well-balanced meals. You will learn practical strategies for portion control and selecting the right combination of foods to avoid blood sugar spikes.

In the third week, you will learn how to tweak your meals according to pre- and post-meal blood glucose levels. Your meal plan will be more effective and personalised, which means you are likely to stick with it.

In the fourth week, you will focus on enhancing the quality of your meal plan and utilizing technology to monitor your blood glucose variation consistently. Through the use of these innovative tools, you will learn how to track your food intake, monitor your blood glucose levels, and identify any patterns or red flags that may have previously gone unnoticed. By the end of this week, you will have developed a deeper understanding of the role of technology in diabetes management and how to leverage it to your advantage.

You will have the tools and knowledge to make informed adjustments to your meal plan and ensure that you stay motivated on your journey towards optimal health.

Figure 7.1: A comprehensive four-week meal planning blueprint

Meal Plan Blueprint			
Week 1: Assess Your Baseline	Week 2: Enhance Your Knowledge	Week 3: Appraise and Fix	Week 4: Rinse and Repeat
• Start a lifestyle journal • Scan your shopping list • Sort your go-to meals	• Know your food groups • Spot the carbs • Fix your plate pattern	• Appraise your meals • Fix your fasting and pre-meal blood glucose • Fix your post-meal blood glucose	• Add super foods • Tweak with continuous glucose monitoring • Lapse, relapse, improvise, and repeat

Week 1: Assess Your Baseline

1. Start a Lifestyle Journal

When I talk to my patients, I always ask, "How do you feel about keeping a journal?" Most of my patients answer, "I've never journaled" and "I'm not sure how it will help."

How will keeping a journal change your life? Writing a journal can help you identify patterns in your diet and activity choices. It can help you to become more mindful and aware of yourself, and to recognise any self-sabotaging tendencies or other issues. By doing this, you can learn to become your own coach and make decisions that are in line with your goals and values. Journaling is truly one of the best self-improvement tools.

You probably think you know what you eat, how much you eat, and what your blood glucose levels are. However, if you track everything you eat and how it impacts your daily blood glucose levels, you'll discover problems you didn't even know existed.

For instance, you might discover that a particular food is causing your blood glucose levels to spike and that you're eating more than you thought you were. By comparing your performance against a benchmark, you can determine how much progress you have made and identify areas that need improvement. Additionally, benchmarking allows you to compare your performance to recommended goals.

A "lifestyle" journal will help you track your eating habits, physical activity, sleep patterns, medications and insulin, and how your blood glucose varies throughout the day. This tracking can provide a level of consciousness and valuable data to help correct intake patterns over time.

For this week, fill out a new sheet each day or keep track of your progress in a notebook, on your laptop, or on your mobile.

You can also use a food weighing scale, measuring spoons, cups, and standard plates to note the portions. This is beneficial because it can be difficult to estimate portion sizes with the naked eye. A food weighing scale can give you an accurate measurement of how much you are consuming. Measuring spoons, cups, and standard plates can also give you an idea of what an appropriate portion size looks like. Additionally, it also helps you to be mindful of how much food you are consuming.

Remember, when recording your observations, be accurate and honest. This is important because if your observations are not accurate and honest, any conclusions you make from them may be misleading or incorrect. Accurate and honest observations are critical for ensuring the reliability of your data.

Self-monitoring of blood glucose (SMBG) is very important toward your progress in glucose control. If you have a glucometer (a device for measuring the glucose concentration in the blood), or any other similar device, check your blood glucose before starting your meal and 2 hours after your meal. Remember to wash your hands thoroughly before your test to avoid errors in the testing. Record your blood glucose levels.

Most people find that taking accountability over time is motivating. This process can offer you ways to become your own counselor and alleviate anxiety.

During a consultation, a patient vividly told me, "I'm so afraid of hyperglycemia that I keep checking every hour and if it rises, I get anxious and sweaty." My advice is don't keep checking your blood glucose constantly. Try not to become anxious or distressed by the variations in your blood glucose levels. This is a process, and you will reach your desired outcome eventually.

When writing your lifestyle journal, commit to leaving out your inner critic. Consider it an experiment where you are gathering helpful information. Keeping a lifestyle journal isn't for you if you struggle with obsessive-compulsive disorder and/or eating disorders. This may cause you to fixate on every detail and become mentally consumed by the numbers. If this sounds like you, stepping away from this tool is important.

The sample lifestyle journal is not intended to be a representative of a healthy lifestyle log, but rather a typical diary of a person with diabetes. It shows how dietary choices, meal timing and physical activity influence blood glucose variation over the course of a day. For instance, drinking fruit juice at 7.30 pm spikes your blood glucose before dinner and stays high afterwards. It is therefore advisable to space out carbohydrate-rich snacks from main meals. A further observation is that higher portions of grains, such as rice, have a marked effect on blood glucose levels (raised from 97 mg/dl to 180 mg/dl). It is, therefore, advisable to control portions of rice.

Table 7.1: Sample Lifestyle Journal Log

Time	8:00 a.m.	9:00 a.m.			Snack	2:00 p.m.			7:30 p.m.	8:00 p.m.			11:30 p.m.
Meal/Task	Fasting	Breakfast			Snack	Lunch			Snack	Dinner			Sleep
Food Eaten, with Portions	tea with milk and 1 tsp sugar	egg sandwich with white bread and 1 cup of tea with milk			nil	rice 2 cups, with fried chicken strips-1 portion, and 1 cup of sautéed vegetables			1 cup of fruit juice	chicken pasta with tomato sauce -1/2 plate and 1 cup grilled vegetables			1 cup of green tea
		Pre-meal	Post-meal			Pre-meal	Post-meal			Pre-meal	Post-meal		
Blood Glucose (mg/dl or mmol/L)	120	110	140			97	180			170	230		
Activity Time					8:00–8:30 a.m.								
Type of Activity, Blood Glucose Pre- and Post- Activity (mg/dl or mmol/l)					Walking-moderate speed Pre-activity 120 Post-activity 110								
Feelings/ Medications/ Insulin/ Hunger-Fullness	Metformin 1,000 mg					very hungry			feeling full				tired

Know Your Targets of Pre-meal and Post-meal Glucose

According to the research of psychologists, neurologists, and other scientists, setting goals pushes us to invest in a target as if we'd already accomplished it. When we set a goal, no matter how small or large, no matter how distant, a part of our brain believes that the desired outcome is an essential part of who we are, so we work toward the goal to fulfill our brain's self-image.

We have discussed blood glucose targets for people with diabetes and prediabetes in Chapter 2. Blood glucose targets are individualised based on several factors, such as the type of diabetes, the duration of diabetes, and the complications of diabetes.

The American Diabetes Association recommends pre-meal blood glucose of 80-130 mg/dl and less than 180 mg/dl post-meal (1-2 hours after beginning the meal).113 Keeping a target of less than 180 mg/dl will help you keep your HbA1c around 7%, but the lower it is, the better it will prevent complications.[114]

If you target your postprandial blood sugar to be less than 140 mg/dl, it will result in an HbA1c of less than or equal to 6%.[115] This is an excellent way to moderate or even reverse diabetes. Record other important numbers, such as your weight, body mass index, blood pressure, HbA1c, blood cholesterol, triglycerides, HDL cholesterol, and LDL cholesterol. You will be pleasantly surprised at how lifestyle changes have positively affected your numbers.

2. Scan Your Shopping List

Did you know that supermarket placement and design tricks can manipulate you to buy certain foods? The fact that you are already influenced by media marketing and environmental cues makes you wonder what retailers could possibly do next. It isn't by accident that the colorful, ultra-processed foods are placed at eye level and easy to access? As though that wasn't enough, your kids are also targets—cereal at the eye level of kids in shopping carts is plastered with cartoon blandishments to get parents to buy it.

We have discussed at length how to identify real food in Chapter 6. Now let's learn how to bring those foods into our kitchen. A supermarket typically carries anywhere from 15,000 to 30,000 food items. No wonder navigating the aisles can feel overwhelming!

Look at your regular grocery list to identify real foods and ultra-processed foods. Analyse how many real food items and ultra-processed foods you choose for every 10 items. Gradually target to reduce 1-2 items each week and replace them with healthier options. This exercise could take a while, but it's worth it. The goal is to change your behaviour forever. This is not about following a fancy diet that shows results for a few months before you revert to your old self.

Here's a sample grocery list that you can review to identify real food and ultra-processed food:

Table 7.2 Sample Grocery List

	Real Food ☺	Ultra-Processed Food ☹	Healthy Add-On
Rice	☺		unpolished rice, millet, quinoa, whole oats, buckwheat
Wheat Flour	☺		whole wheat flour
Instant Noodles		☹	pasta, whole wheat pasta
Breakfast Cereal		☹	steel-cut oats porridge, whole wheat chapati, homemade cereal wraps
Cookies		☹	homemade healthy cookies
Frozen Vegetables	☺		fresh vegetables

Cheese	☺		cottage cheese, feta cheese, ricotta
Soda		☹	sparkling water
Nuts	☺		fresh mixed nuts
Apples	☺		all seasonal fruits
Chicken/ Sausages		☹	fresh organic chicken

One tip before you head out for your weekly grocery shopping is to shop after a meal or have a snack before the trip. When you are emotional and craving food, you are more likely to pick your indulgence over rational decision-making. If you are eager to eat your favorite snack, pick it up and portion it slowly. Locally made snacks might also be a suitable alternative to highly processed snacks. After all, isn't enjoying a scoop of your favourite flavour at the local ice cream shop more fun than eating a pint of ice cream while standing over the sink at home?

3. Sort Your Go-To Meals

Let's face it, there are times when you feel too tired or lazy to cook, and dining out or ordering food is the most tempting indulgence. It's important for you to be prepared for such teasers by having a list of meals that you can rely on.

Research a few go-to take aways so that you know which is the healthiest option for that night that you just can't be bothered cooking and want to order in. For example, Thai tends to be healthier than Chinese, and you could make your own portion of brown rice to make it even better. Middle eastern choices are healthier if loaded with lots of fresh salads.

Stay inspired by exploring healthy cookbooks, cooking shows, vlogs, and blogs to discover new recipes. Create a go-to list consisting of five main courses, four salads, three snacks, two sandwiches, and one dessert. Keep your fridge stocked with the necessary ingredients for these recipes and periodically update your go-to list with new options while removing any you no longer enjoy.

Studies have shown that the most common barrier to adherence to healthy eating is the lack of healthy options, time constraints, and laziness.[116] Having a go-to option that's healthy and prepared beforehand will make the journey easier and more enjoyable. Refer to Chapter 6 for tips and tricks and to the index for recipes.

Week 2: Enhance Your Knowledge
1. Know Your Food Groups

The key to healthy eating is to enjoy a variety of foods from all the food groups in the right proportion and the right combination. This will ensure that you receive all the needed nutrients and that you don't deprive yourself of the natural flavours of life.

Do you remember learning about food groups in school? Here's a back-to-basics refresher lesson on the food groups. The five food groups are fruits, vegetables, grains, protein foods, and dairy. You will use these five groups as building blocks for a wholesome, healthy meal. While oils aren't a food group, they are part of a healthy eating pattern because they are a major source of essential fatty acids and vitamin E.

Each food group includes a variety of similar foods in nutritional makeup, and each group plays an extremely significant role in an overall healthy eating pattern. Some food groups are further broken down into subgroups to emphasise foods that are particularly helpful for keeping your blood glucose at optimum levels. Food groups simplify meal planning by focusing on foods instead of on nutrients; for example, we can identify good carbohydrates and mix them with good protein and fat for a meal.

Table 7.3 Food Groups, Subgroups, Glycaemic Index, and Sample Foods

Food Group	Subgroup	High Carbohydrate Source (yes/no)	Glycaemic Index (high/medium/low)	Sample Foods
Grains	Whole grains, millets	yes	low to medium	wholewheat bread, brown rice, oatmeal, millet, popcorn
	Refined grains	yes	high	noodles, croissants, muffins, tortillas, white bread

Vegetables	Non-starchy vegetables	no	low	green vegetables, red peppers, tomatoes, zucchini, okra, eggplant, carrots
	Starchy vegetables	yes	high	potatoes, corn, green peas, sweet potato, beets
Fruits	Whole fruit	yes	low to medium	apples, oranges, cherries, bananas, peaches
	Fruit juice	yes	high	fresh fruit juice, no sugar fruit juice, fruit nectar
Protein	Plant-based protein	yes	low	beans, lentils, chickpeas, soya bean
	Lan and red meat	no	low	beef, lamb, poultry, egg, fish

| Milk | Cheese | no | low | slice cheese; cream cheese; fresh, soft, and hard cheese |
| | Milk and yoghurt | yes | low | low-fat, no-fat, full-fat milk; and yoghurt |

Source: Adapted from the 2020-2025 Dietary Guidelines for Americans.[117]

2. Spot the Carbs

Carbohydrate-containing food groups include grains, fruits, milk and yoghurt, beans/legumes, and starchy vegetables.

Remember that the body breaks down simple carbohydrates quickly, causing a sharp rise in blood glucose. To recap simple carbohydrates are available in fruits and milk as glucose, fructose, sucrose, and lactose. In addition, all the sugars and sugar substitutes found in processed and refined sugars, such as candy, table sugar, syrups, and soft drinks, are rich in simple carbohydrates. Complex carbohydrates are found in grains, beans/legumes, and vegetables.

The meat and cheese group doesn't contribute to carbohydrates in your meal, which means they don't have a direct influence on your blood glucose but have an indirect influence by increasing insulin resistance through saturated fat (refer to Chapter 2).

Hidden Sources of Carbohydrates

By now I am sure you can quickly name the biggest carb offenders, like rice, pasta and bread but you rarely think beyond that in search of sources of carbohydrates in your food. The shocking truth is that carbs aren't just lurking in obvious places; they're hiding out in seemingly innocent foods, like coleslaw, chicken nuggets, sauces, and foods labeled as sugar-free.

When shopping for packaged food, look at the food label for the list of ingredients. These ingredients are listed in order of weight, beginning with the ingredient that weighs the most and ending with the ingredient that weighs the least.

There are many different names for sugar—honey, agave, cane sugar, coconut sugar, maple syrup, corn syrup, or fruit sugar, to name a few. One of the easiest ways to recognise sugar on a food label is by seeing the "-ose" suffix. When you find words that end in -ose, there's a high chance they are sugar.

Sugars ending in -ose include sucrose, maltose, dextrose, fructose, glucose, galactose, lactose, high fructose corn syrup, and glucose solids. A helpful rule of thumb is to scan the first three ingredients and ensure they don't say sugar or sugar substitutes.

3. Fix Your Plate Pattern

"Healthy eating" can take many forms, depending on whom you ask. Everyone seems to have an opinion about the healthiest way to eat, whether they are healthcare professionals, wellness influencers, co-workers, or family. Furthermore, many diets claim high levels of health, sometimes without any evidence.

A healthy lifestyle should be enjoyable, not stressful. Healthy eating doesn't have to be that complicated. No single diet works for everyone, and eating habits will evolve over time based on our unique health status, age, gender, and lifestyle factors.

Making a healthy plate is the most important but simplest step toward living on a healthy meal plan.

Step 1: Right Combination

Make a meal with a combination of food items from the groups of grains, proteins, and vegetables, especially during your main meals, such as lunch and dinner. Fruits and dairy can make great snacks between meals or as breakfast.

Grain products are foods made from wheat, rice, oats, corn, barley, or other cereal grain. Rice, bread, pasta, oatmeal, grits, chapati and tortillas are examples of grain products. Proteins include animal and plant-based sources. However, lean meat and plant-based sources are recommended. Have a variety of vegetables in order to provide your body with the nutrients it needs and also, so you don't get bored!

Step 2: Enhance Fibre

You can control your blood glucose spikes and enhance the quality of your food by choosing foods high in dietary fibre. Dietary fibre can keep you full, help you lose weight, lower your LDL cholesterol, and improve your general health.

When you choose whole grains with high fibre content, you can lower your risk for type 2 diabetes, and if you already have diabetes, they can slow your blood glucose absorption. Vegetables like gourds, sweet potato, and cauliflower; green vegetables like kale, spinach, and lettuce; and plant-based proteins like green beans, lentils, chickpeas, and nuts are excellent sources of soluble fibre that reduce the post-meal spike in blood glucose.

Step 3: The Right Proportion

Have a close look at your weekly food journal to understand your proportions. Grains, vegetables, and protein should all be included in your meals in the correct amounts. Have a close look at your plate and identify the proportion of grains, vegetables, and protein. Your ideal proportion of grains, vegetables and proteins should be 1:2:1 (25%, 50%, 25%). Understanding this proportion for each food group will help you move your glucose levels.

Nevertheless, if your plate resembles stage 1, you should gradually move to stage 2 and ultimately reach stage 3 to achieve the best control of your glucose levels.

See the following figures for a typical transition in plate patterns.

The 3rd C - Create Your Own Meal Plan

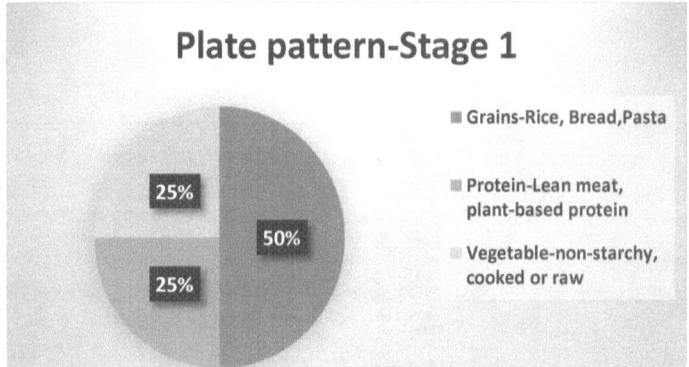

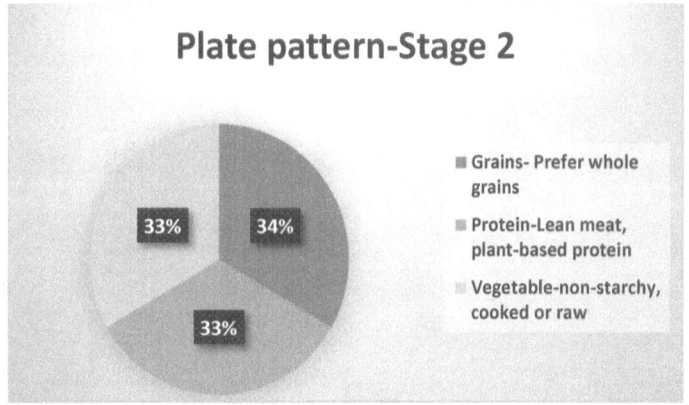

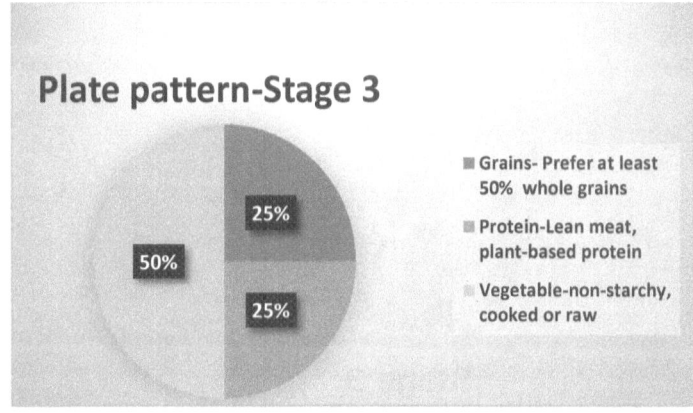

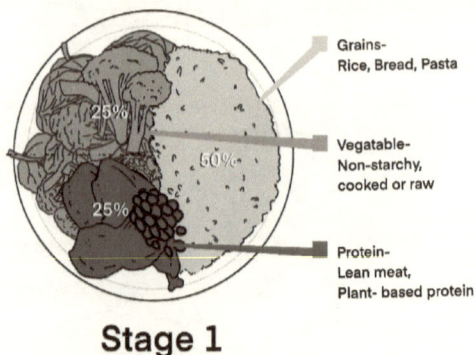

Stage 1

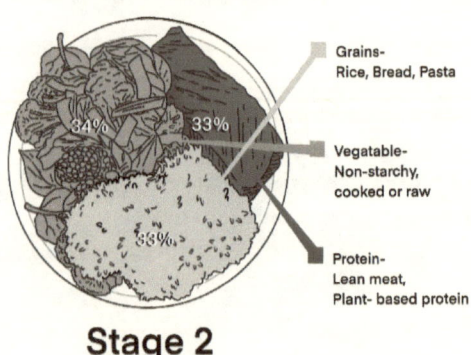

Stage 2

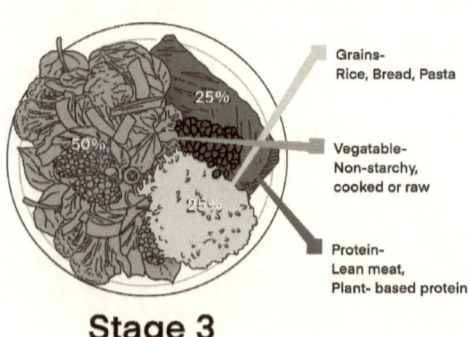

Stage 3

Rule of 1:2 (Grains: Vegetables)

This rule represents the portions of grains to vegetables in your main meals (lunch and dinner).

Raw vegetables:

Have a ratio of 1:2 (grains: vegetables), when measuring raw vegetables. For every portion of grains, double the portion of vegetables (raw) in volume or weight. For instance, if you are adding one cup of grains, have two cups of vegetables.

Cooked vegetables:

However, if you are eating cooked vegetables, you add 1 cup of cooked vegetables for 1 cup of grains. It is because 2 cups of raw vegetables are equivalent to 1 cup of cooked vegetables. To put it simply, when eating cooked vegetables, have a ratio of 1:1 (grains: vegetables)

Combination of raw and cooked vegetables:

In a meal with grains, raw salad and cooked vegetables, keep a 1:1:1 ratio (Grain: Raw vegetable: Cooked vegetable).

Example of how to make the proportion of grains and vegetables:

1. 1 cup of boiled brown rice with 1 cup of vegetable curry/ vegetable stir fry, or 1 cup of boiled pasta cooked with 2 cups of mixed vegetables.
2. 150g boiled brown rice and 300g salad, OR 150g boiled brown rice with 150g cooked vegetables (since cooking reduces the volume to half of raw, 1 cup raw vegetable is ½ cup cooked vegetable),

3. A plate of 150g cooked quinoa, 150g green salad and 75g vegetable stew.

Example of a complete meal plate:

- 1 cup boiled rice, 1 portion grilled chicken, and 2 cups salad.
- Whole grain bread sandwiched with 1/2 portion of chicken and 1/2 cup of vegetables sautéed.
- 1 cup boiled rice, 1 cup lentil curry, and 1 cup vegetable soup.
- Oat porridge made from rolled oats (1/2 cup), grilled chicken (1 portion), and vegetables (1 cup).

Tip: Keep fruit, milk, and yoghurt for snacks between meals for now.

Step 4: Right Portions (Quantity)

The portion of food you choose has a direct influence on your calorie intake. To get started, determine your calorie target. Do you want to lose weight or maintain your weight? Next, use a calorie calculator (e.g., the Mifflin–St. Jeor formula) to estimate the number of daily calories. Note that fewer than 1,200 to 1,500 kcal/day for women and 1,500 to 1,800 kcal/day for men generally aren't recommended because you may not get enough nutrients.

Calories are derived from different foods in certain amounts. Reading several research papers and working with thousands of people with diabetes in this region, I have concluded that the healthiest option is a *Mediterranean diet* focused on *plant-based, minimally processed foods*. The evidence is overwhelming that these dietary choices not only prevent diabetes but also manage

The 3rd C - Create Your Own Meal Plan

blood glucose, lipid profiles, and blood pressure, and prevent complications of diabetes.

Now you know how many calories you should consume in a day. But you don't eat calories, you eat food. You have learnt that foods are divided into food groups, so now we can put the pieces together. Let's measure the size of food items you can consume in a day and in a week in each food group in terms of servings.

Table 7.4 The recommended daily servings from each food group based on the calorie intake.

Food Group	Subgroup	Serving Size	Servings Per Day (1400-1600 kcal)	Servings Per Day (1800-2000 kcal)
Grains (ounce / day)	whole grains, millets	1 slice bread, ½ cup dry cereal, ⅓ cup cooked rice, pasta, or cereal	2-3	3-4
	refined grains		2-3	3-4
Vegetables (cup /day)	non-starchy vegetables	1 cup salad, ½ cup cooked vegetables	3-4	4-6
	starchy vegetables		1	1

Fruits (cup /day)	whole Fruit	1 medium fruit, ¼ cup dried fruit, ½ cup fresh, frozen, or canned fruit, ½ cup fruit juice	1-2	2-3
Protein (ounce / day)	plant-based protein	⅓ cup beans, ⅓ cup cooked lentils or baked beans	½-1	½-1
	lean and red meat	30g cooked meats, poultry, or fish, 1 egg	1-2	2-3
Dairy (cup /day)	cheese	28 g cheese	0-½	½
	milk and yoghurt	1 cup milk or yoghurt	1-2	1-2
Nuts (ounce / week)	fresh nuts and seeds	⅓ cup nuts, 2 tbsp peanut butter, 2 tbsp seeds	2	4

Oil (tsp/day)		1 teaspoon vegetable oil, olive oil	3-4	4-5
Sweet/ Savoury Snacks (ounce / week)		30 g chocolate/ small pack savory, 2 biscuits	≤ 2	≤ 3

One ounce is 28 grams (~30 grams). Adapted from the Dietary Guidelines for Americans 2020-2025 and the American Diabetes Association Nutrition position paper 2019.

Understanding what and how much to eat can be a complex task. Discuss with your registered dietitian for assistance, if needed, based on your preferences, and eating habits.

Eating smaller portions can be challenging for most, especially at first. Try these tricks to help you control your portions: eat slowly, be mindful of what you are eating, have your salad first before the main meal, don't starve before you eat, and use smaller plates to serve.

Week 3: Appraise and Fix

1. Appraise your Meals

Remember that your journal is for your eyes only. With even the faintest thought that others will read your writing, you will start to self-edit. Check if you have filled out honest, objective information without fearing judgment. The built-in food journal will make you mindful of what you eat, how much you eat, and how you feel before, during, and after you eat. A research study on people with diabetes and prediabetes has shown that participants who tracked their food intake for at least five days a week lost an additional 4.5 kg of weight compared to those who rarely tracked their food. A research study by Ingels et al in 2017 on people with......

Ask these questions to spot red flags

Assess your meal pattern:

a. How many meals and snacks do you consume each day?
b. Are you eating two to three meals every day or skipping meals and having one big meal? Do you graze all day long or enjoy only main meals?
c. How frequently do you eat food from restaurants and takeaways?

Assess variety:

a. Are you choosing food from all the food groups (grains, protein, milk, vegetables, fruits)?
b. Are you including a variety of foods or eating the same foods repeatedly?
c. Do you include all colours of vegetables and a variety of, or limited choices?

Assess hunger:

a. Which time of the day are you most hungry, and are you indulging in calorie-dense food out of hunger or desire?
b. Are you choosing food out of liking or availability?
c. How frequently do you eat food from restaurants and takeaways?

Assess the quality and quantity of carbohydrates:

a. Do you consume more simple or complex carbohydrates?
b. Can you possibly switch simple carbohydrates to complex carbohydrates?
c. What's the quality of grains?
d. Are they whole or refined grains?
e. What is the size of your food portions?

Assess the meal pattern:

a. Are you choosing real food with portions of grains, vegetables, and protein?
b. Do whole grains make up to 50% of your total grains?
c. Do you eat more plant-based proteins or red meat?
d. Is the ratio of vegetables to grains 1:2?

Are You Snack-Smart?

Snacks are foods eaten between main meals. People snack for many reasons, such as they are feeling hungry, having low energy, craving a particular food; or they feel stressed, anxious, or bored. Snacking can get you into a health trap unless you know how to choose your snacks smartly.

Typical snack foods can harm your health, as they are easy-to-find, ultra-processed foods high in sodium, unhealthy fats, and refined carbohydrates. The good news is that, when done thoughtfully, you can reap the benefits of snacking. Snacking is the best window to introduce fruits, milk, and yoghurt to your meal plan, as they are sources of good carbohydrates, but adding them to the main meal will increase the carbohydrate load of the meals. The best way is to space snacks between meals.

My patients often ask me, "Can and should I have a snack between meals if I have diabetes?" The simple answer is, if you manage your diabetes with healthy eating of three meals per day, physical activity, and/or certain types of diabetes pills, such as metformin, you may not need to eat a snack.

On the other hand, if you take insulin or diabetes pills called sulfonylureas, snacking may be recommended to help you prevent low blood glucose. Your healthcare team can help determine if snacking is a good choice for you. Another factor to keep in mind is your daily schedule. It is recommended that you shouldn't go for more than 5 to 6 hours without eating if you have diabetes.

For example, if you eat breakfast at 7 a.m., and lunch isn't until 2 p.m., having a late-morning healthy snack can keep your blood glucose levels steady and keep your hunger pangs in check, too. On the other hand, if you dine at 8 p.m. and go to bed at 10 p.m., you probably don't need a bedtime snack (but you may need a snack depending on your blood sugar levels).

Now that you count your carbohydrates, a general guideline for choosing a healthy snack is to aim for about 15 grams to no more than 30 grams of carbs. Smart snacks include a handful of nuts with green tea, a hard-boiled egg, raw veggies dipped in low-fat cottage cheese or hummus or spiced yoghurt, whole grain toast with nut butter, fresh fruit, a cup of plant-based milk with a handful of nuts, and a cup of plain yoghurt or milk.

Snack on Fresh Fruit or Fruit Juice?

A common question my patients always ask me is, "Can I have fruits? They are sweet and have sugars like fructose and glucose, right?" Yes, you can have fruits; however, choose the portion size and the timing of when you eat them. Fruits are great sources of nutrients, fibre, and the fruit sugar "fructose." Nature is the best provider, as it has packed fruits with the sweetness of glucose and fructose, but it also provides antidotes to this sweetness, which include fibre, antioxidants, and phytonutrients. These antidotes nullify the effect of fructose (Petta, 2013).

On the contrary, large population studies have reported a protective action of fruits on the risk of diabetes and glycemic control in people with diabetes (Nichola, 2021). My cross-sectional study on 843 people with diabetes in the United Arab Emirates showed that fresh fruit intake improved glycemic control. Meanwhile, even weekly, fruit juices, sugar-sweetened beverages, and soda consumption significantly deteriorated glucose control (Sadiya, 2019). This means that consuming fruits is not only harmless but is actually helpful in managing your diabetes and preventing complications.

Although juice and smoothie companies state that their products contain only natural sugars, fruit and fruit juice are not equivalent. Even if you consume the same number of calories from whole fruit and juice, the metabolic effects are very different. Metabolically speaking, fruit juice is much more like soda than whole fruit. As shown below, different forms of orange can affect your blood glucose differently.

Table 7.5 Nutritional difference between fresh orange, orange juice and orange soda

	Medium Orange	Orange Juice (1 cup)	Orange Soda (1 cup)
Sugar (grams)	15	22	30
Fibre	++ 3	+/-	-
Vitamins	++	++	-
Satiety (fullness)	++	+/-	-
Effect on Blood Glucose	a slow, controlled rise in blood glucose	rapid blood sugar spike and fall	rapid blood sugar spike and fall

Hence a smart snack choice will be fresh, seasonal, colourful fruits high in antioxidants and dietary fibre like berries, oranges, apples, plums, papaya, kiwi, guava, and pears and smaller portions of high glycemic index sweetened fruits like mangoes, bananas, jackfruit, and grapes. Juices could be replaced with whole fruits, ice cream sundaes could be replaced with frozen yoghurt, and soda could be replaced with sparkling water with lemon and mint.

2. Fix Your Fasting and Pre-Meal Blood Glucose
Fasting Blood Glucose

When you fast for a long time, your body needs glucose for energy; this is drawn from the reserved glucose as glycogen in the liver. The hormone "insulin" is responsible for this action. If a person doesn't have diabetes, their body will produce insulin to rebalance the increased glucose levels; this is reflected in the fasting blood glucose of less than 100 mg/dl (5.6 mmol/l).

However, people with diabetes either don't produce enough insulin to rebalance their blood glucose (beta cell dysfunction) or their body can't use the insulin effectively (insulin resistance). Hence their fasting blood glucose is elevated more than people without diabetes. The American Diabetes Association recommends fasting blood glucose between 100-125 g/dl indicated prediabetes and 125 mg/dl and higher indicated diabetes[2]. If you are diagnosed with diabetes, your optimum fasting blood glucose goal should be:

- **The American Diabetes Association recommends goals within a 70-130 mg/dl (3.9-7.2 mmol/l) range**[2]
- **The American Association of Clinical Endocrinologists suggests a target at <110 mg/dl (6.1 mmol/l).** [118]
- **The International Diabetes Federation suggests a target of < 100 mg/dl (5.5 mmol/l).**[119]

However, your target fasting blood glucose should be discussed with your treating physician.

Low fasting blood glucose is common for people with type 1 diabetes and can occur in people with type 2 diabetes taking insulin or certain medications. Talk to your diabetes care team about your own blood glucose targets and what level is too low for you.

While you are on your 5C journey, be patient and monitor your fasting blood glucose over the next four weeks. As you begin to change your meal portions and proportions, meal timings, sleeping patterns, and activity routine, you will likely notice a steady decline in your fasting blood glucose levels.

Pre-Meal Blood Glucose

It's ideal for testing your pre-meal blood glucose when at least 3 to 4 hours have passed without snacks between meals. For example, if you ate breakfast at 8.00 a.m. and lunch at 1.00 p.m. without any snacks between 11.00 a.m. and 1.00 p.m., then you can be assured that this pre-meal blood glucose level has no overlap effect from a previous meal.

If you are taking rapid-acting insulin with your meals, pre-meal tests are a good way of seeing whether you have injected the right units of insulin dose for your previous meal. If you have injected too little insulin, you will see your pre-meal results are higher than they should be before your next meal. If you have injected too much insulin, your test results will be too low before your next meal. If you have questions about insulin dosing, write them down and discuss them with your healthcare team.

If you take oral medications, your pre-meal tests will reveal how well your body handled your previous meal with the assistance of your medications. Having high pre-meal results may indicate that the carbohydrates you consumed in a previous meal were too much or that your medication is inadequate.

The American Diabetes Association recommends a pre-meal target of 80-130 mg/dl (4.4-7.2 mmol/l), while the National Institute for Health and Care Excellence guidelines recommend 72-126 mg/dl (4-7 mmol/l).[120, 121]

3. Fix Your Post-Meal Blood Glucose

Your fasting blood glucose doesn't inform you about how good or damaging your diet is. Post-meal or "postprandial," meaning glucose in the blood after the meal, gives you information about how your body can manage glucose after a meal. The post-meal peaks are temporary high blood glucose levels that occur soon after eating. The blood glucose level rises after eating and falls back to normal within 2 hours, even for people without diabetes. A post-meal glucose peak of up to 140 mg/dL (7.8 mmol/L) is considered normal if you don't have diabetes or prediabetes. However, in people with diabetes, this rise is too steep, and the fall back to pre-meal levels is often too slow. Even though these peaks are temporary, a series of them over time means that your blood has been exposed to higher glucose levels for a longer period.

This results in more caramelization of haemoglobin molecules, thus a higher HbA1c level. Your HbA1c test result reflects your average blood glucose level for all times of day (before and after meals) over the past 2 to 3 months, with the more recent weeks influencing the result more than earlier weeks. Numerous studies have strongly indicated that a higher HbA1c increases the risk of complications of diabetes affecting the heart, eyes, nerves, and kidneys.[122]

I have frequently heard patients say, "I check my blood glucose before breakfast, and it's normal." They believe this indicates their blood sugar is under control, so they can relax on diet and on lifestyle. In reality, this is less than half the puzzle as the post-meal peaks are the most influential factor that affects your HbA1c.

So, exactly how high is too high after a meal?

There's no universal consensus on this issue. The American Diabetes Association recommends keeping blood glucose below 180 mg/dl 1 to 2 hours after the start of a meal[2]. The American Association of Clinical Endocrinologists and the International Diabetes Federation recommend keeping it below 140 mg/dl after eating.[123, 124] The NICE guidelines of the United Kingdom recommend below 153 mg/dl (8.5 mmol/L) for people with type 2 diabetes and less than 162 mg/dl (9 mmol/l) for people with type 1 diabetes.[125]

However, the post-meal peak depends on your pre-meal blood glucose.

What I mean by this is that for 2 people with the same post-meal reading of 180, if person A has a pre-meal level of 80 and person B has a pre meal level of 120 then the rise is higher in person A.

As of now, we don't have a consensus regarding the acceptable amount of rise. Discuss with your physician/healthcare provider and identify the most appropriate targets based on your type of diabetes, insulin use, children versus adults, and complications associated with diabetes.

Here are some fascinating research studies showcasing how making small changes in your meals can effectively reduce post-meal glucose spikes.

i. Portion Control

Most of us "cheat" when talking about what we eat. Sometimes this is intentional—we don't want people to know—but mostly it is unintentional, we forget the piece of cheese we snuck out of the fridge when making a cup of tea, or we underestimate the portion size we actually ate.

And if you are hungry, research suggests that you will miscalculate portion sizes to a greater degree than you would after eating a meal.[126] Besides helping you control your blood glucose levels, learning portion control also helps you lose weight.

It isn't always easy to get your portion sizes right; this can make managing your weight and blood glucose levels more difficult.

You can use a food weighing scale for clearer accuracy. For instance, when you measure a portion of rice by plate or spoon and then check by weight, there will most likely be a variation of 10-20%, and mostly it's an overestimation.[127] A common misestimate is bread. The recipe says, 'A slice of bread' but all bread slices are not equal! If it has a food label that is easier, but traditional or homemade bread doesn't have a label.

In my practice, I use a simple estimation that involves weighing the bread and estimating half of the weight as carbohydrates. For example, if your bread weighs 120 grams, it's estimated to contain 60 grams of carbohydrates.

Measuring all your food for a period will give you enough experience to be able to eventually just eyeball your foods to get your portions right.

Your lifestyle journal will help you gauge the right portions for you depending on your pre- and post-meal glucose levels. If you take your medications as prescribed and the difference between your pre-meal and post-meal glucose is around 40 mg/dl, your medications and your glucose from the meal are optimum.

However, if the difference is 80 mg/dl or more, this indicates higher portions of carbohydrates in the meal or inadequate medication.

ii. Quality of Carbohydrates

By now, you are aware of simple and complex carbohydrates. Replacing simple with complex is the first go-to solution. Ultra-processed foods are loaded with simple carbohydrates. Switching to minimally processed foods reduces the post-meal peak.

Adding sources of dietary fibre is another simple technique to lessen the post-meal glucose spike. The main sources of dietary fibre are whole grains, beans and pulses, and vegetables. If you adhere to the plate pattern, you get most of it right.

Dietary fibre is effective at delaying gastric emptying (movement of food from the stomach to the intestines), slowing digestion, and reducing the post-meal peak of both glucose and triglycerides.

An interesting study published in a nutrition journal of 17 participants with diabetes reported that adding pinto beans, red kidney beans, and black beans to the rice portion significantly plateaus the post-meal peak.[128]

Another study from Singapore showed that the post-meal peak to white rice with a chicken breast, ground nut oil, and vegetables was significantly lower than to white rice alone. The glycemic index of pure white rice was 96; whereas, combined with a chicken breast, ground nut oil, and vegetables, it was 50.[129]

iii. Protein and Fats

Sources of lean protein, plant-based protein, and unsaturated fats have been shown to reduce glucose spikes after meals due to a slow digestive process (gastric delaying). Lean-quality protein has been shown to reduce post-meal glucose spike and improve satiety (O'Keefe, 2008). Recent studies also show that nuts like almonds, pistachios, or peanuts, when eaten with high glycemic index carbohydrates, such as white bread or mashed potatoes, will reduce the post-meal glucose rise by approximately 30 to 50%.[130] A slice of whole-grain bread with nut butter could be a good choice for a healthy breakfast.

A mixture of vinegar and olive oil is the traditional salad dressing used in the Mediterranean diet and is also shown to reduce the post-meal glucose peak. Recent studies show that 1 to 2 tablespoons of vinegar when added to a meal containing high glycemic index foods, such as white bread or white rice, lowers post-meal glucose by 25 to 35%.[131]

Vinegar significantly reduces post-meal glycaemia, because acetic acid slows gastric emptying and thus delays carbohydrate absorption and improves satiety. Another study in diabetes reported that adding extra virgin olive oil to a high glycemic index food could plateau the post-meal glucose peak by almost 50%.[132]

Therefore, the plate pattern will help you reach the peak when you mix grains, lean meats, and vegetables in assigned proportions.

iv. Meal Sequencing

In the last decade, there has been some interesting research on how meal sequencing (the order in which you eat fibre, protein, and carbohydrates) influences your post-meal glucose. A pilot study published in 2015 showed that consuming proteins and vegetables first, followed by carbohydrate portions, significantly reduces the post-meal peak in people with type 2 diabetes.[133]

v. Activity and Sleeping Patterns

Post-meal physical exercise is safe and effective in bringing down the glucose spike. Walking for even 15 to 20 minutes after eating results in a reduced glucose spike.[134] How does exercise do this? Simply put, exercise acutely increases glucose uptake in skeletal muscle, and it does it immediately. (Goodyear, 1998).

The optimal timing for post-meal exercise has been suggested to be 30 minutes after the start of a meal.[135] This is because peak post-meal glucose values typically occur within 90 minutes, and initiating exercise during this time window will lessen glucose spikes, protecting the walls of the blood cells from sticky glucose concentrations.[136, 137]

Physical activity is important for everyone with diabetes. Managing glucose levels with any form of exercise is possible once you understand your personal patterns (doing regular blood glucose checks and keeping a workout log can help) and make adjustments that make sense to you and your lifestyle.

Sleep also plays an important role in maintaining healthy blood glucose levels. (This is discussed in detail in Chapter 6.). Even partial sleep deprivation over one night increases insulin resistance, which can, in turn, increase blood sugar levels. And just as sleep affects blood sugar levels, blood sugar levels may also impact sleep quality. Vicious circle, right?

Keep in mind that blood glucose results can trigger strong feelings and leave you upset, confused, frustrated, angry, or sad. It's easy to use your level numbers to judge yourself. Remember though that tracking your blood glucose levels is simply a way to know how well your diabetes care plan is working and whether that plan may need to change.

Week 4: Rinse and Repeat

1. Add Superfoods

"Superfood" is a term used by many food and beverage companies to promote a food thought to have health benefits; however, there's no official definition of the word by the Food and Drug Administration (FDA). The list of foods below is rich in nutrients essential for the optimum health of a person with diabetes. These nutrients are good for overall health and may also help prevent disease.

Omega-3 Essential Fat

Omega-3 fats are essential fats because they cannot be synthesised by the body and must be supplemented through food. These fats produce hormone-like substances called prostaglandins that are essential for several vital functions like reducing the stickiness of the blood, controlling blood cholesterol, reducing inflammation, and improving immune functions.

The best sources of omega-3 fats are fish like mackerel, salmon, herring, and sardines, and plant sources like flax seeds, chia seeds, and walnuts.

Fish

Fish is an excellent source of high-quality protein and is low in saturated fat. Some fish contain omega-3 fats that may help combat heart disease and inflammation. Fish high in these healthy fats is sometimes called "fatty fish." Salmon, herring, sardines, mackerel, trout, and tuna are well-known examples of fatty fish. The American Diabetes Association Standards of Medical Care in Diabetes recommends eating fish (mainly fatty fish) twice per week for people with diabetes.[138]

However, stay away from fish with higher levels of mercury like shark, swordfish, king mackerel, marlin, and fresh tuna, especially if you are pregnant or breastfeeding or have children younger than 11 years old.[139]

Flaxseeds

Extensive research studies have shown that flaxseeds consumed daily at a low dose of 13g help in decreasing fasting blood glucose in prediabetic and diabetic patients.[140] Flaxseed and its components have an anti-diabetic effect. Glycemic control is improved by flaxseeds and its compounds. Another study was performed in 2009 on 20 people with type 2 diabetes, where they were regularly fed chapatti that contained 5 grams of flaxseed and 25 grams of wheat flour for 3 months and compared to the control group that was nondiabetic. Results showed a considerable reduction in blood glucose levels. Besides lowering fasting blood glucose, flaxseeds have been shown to significantly reduce the post-meal glucose spike.[141]

Chia Seeds

Chia seeds are small black seeds rich in oils and omega-3 fats, antioxidants, fibre, and magnesium. They may help reduce the risk of type 2 diabetes and diabetes complications. Research trials on people with type 2 diabetes showed that consuming 40 grams of chia seeds incorporated into food for 12 weeks could lower systolic blood pressure significantly. In addition, adding 31.5 grams of chia seeds to meals could significantly reduce the post-meal glucose spike. These findings affirm that chia seeds don't act alone to benefit human health but may contribute to disease prevention when incorporated as part of a varied plant-rich diet and other healthy lifestyle behaviors.[142]

Here are some tips for adding flaxseeds and chia seeds to your diet:

They are best absorbed when freshly ground and sprinkled on your meals. If you have a coffee grinder you can use it to grind equal portions of both seeds, place them in a glass jar, and store them in the fridge away from light, heat, and oxygen. Simply adding one heaped tablespoon to your meal guarantees a good quality daily intake of omega-3 fats.

You can also safely add other sources of omega-3 fats to this mixture, such as walnuts or pumpkin seeds.

Antioxidant-Rich Foods

The body generates free radicals as a by-product of normal processes in cells, and because of other factors such as tobacco smoke, ultraviolet rays, and air pollution. Free radicals are unstable compounds, and in high doses, they increase the risk of diabetes, heart disease, and cancer. Antioxidants are molecules that fight free radicals in your body.

Your body has its own antioxidant defenses to keep free radicals in check. Adding dietary antioxidants to your diet can strengthen your body's defense against these diseases.

Many nutrient-dense foods are rich in antioxidants, including certain types of berries, nuts, and vegetables. These foods have also been linked to other health benefits and may protect against chronic disease.

Plant-based and animal-based foods contain antioxidants, although plant-based foods have up to 100 times more antioxidant content than animal-based foods (mean antioxidant activity 11.57 mmol/g vs. 0.1 mmol/g).[143]

The simplest approach to supercharging your diet with antioxidants is to consume plenty of brightly coloured fruits and vegetables along with whole grains, seeds, nuts, beans, and legumes. You might have noticed that the types of foods listed are the same ones recommended to control diabetes.

Here are some superfoods that are loaded with antioxidants:

Berries

Which are your favourites—blueberries, strawberries, acai berries, blackberries, cherries, or another variety? Regardless, they are all packed with antioxidants, vitamins, and fibre. Berries are the healthiest fruits, and they can be a great option to satisfy your sweet tooth. They provide the added benefit of coloured plant pigments rich in phytonutrients like resveratrol, anthocyanins and lycopene, with vitamin C, vitamin K, manganese, potassium, and fibre.

Coffee and Tea

Coffee and tea, preferably without milk, creamer, sugar, or sweetener, are considered two of the healthiest beverages. These superfoods are not only sources of high concentrations of antioxidants, but they are also loaded with caffeine. But there is a downside!

Worldwide, the predominant sources of caffeine are coffee, tea, colas, energy drinks, and cocoa (chocolate). Have you ever wondered why you get hooked on drinking coffee, particularly in the morning? Is it because coffee increases your energy and alertness, or is it because it relieves the withdrawal symptoms of coffee (source of caffeine)?

Dr. Peter Rogers, a professor of psychiatry and pharmacology at Vanderbilt University, found that regular coffee drinkers need caffeine to return to their normal state of alertness and avoid the side effects of caffeine withdrawal, such as headaches.

If you aren't a coffee drinker, you get the same alertness from your own natural stimulants—dopamine and adrenalin. In other words, drinking coffee relieves the symptoms of caffeine withdrawal. It's addictive.[144]

Coffee is an intricate mixture of more than a thousand chemicals. What defines a cup of coffee is the type of coffee bean, roasting method, grind amount, and brewing method. Human responses to coffee or caffeine can also vary substantially across individuals. The more caffeine you consume, the more your body and brain become insensitive to their own natural stimulants. You then need more external stimulation to feel normal.

Although the ingestion of caffeine can increase blood sugar in the short-term, long-term studies have shown that habitual coffee drinkers have a lower risk of developing type 2 diabetes compared with nondrinkers.[145] The polyphenols and minerals, such as magnesium, in coffee may improve the effectiveness of insulin and glucose metabolism in the body.

In a meta-analysis of 45,335 people with type 2 diabetes followed for up to 20 years, an association was found between increasing cups of coffee and a lower risk of developing diabetes. Compared with no coffee, the decreased risk ranged from 8% with 1 cup a day to 33% with 6 cups a day. The benefits of caffeine-containing coffee were slightly greater than those of decaffeinated coffee.[146]

An umbrella review of 17 meta-analyses suggested that coffee consumption seems generally safe with an intake of 3 to 4 cups per day.[147] However, the extra calories, sugar, and saturated fat in a coffee house beverage loaded with whipped cream and flavoured syrup might offset any health benefits found in a basic black coffee.

You don't have to start drinking coffee if you don't already or to increase the amount you currently drink, as there are many other dietary strategies to improve your health.

Black tea, green tea, and white tea are all made from the leaves of the same tea shrub, with different levels of processing. White tea is the least processed of all teas. In contrast, herbal teas can come from any herb or plant but are not from the tea plant.

The tea shrub is loaded with phytonutrients with high antioxidant activity; however, processing significantly reduces these antioxidants. White and green tea is less processed than black tea, so they are more beneficial. Studies have shown some promising results of matcha green tea compounds and cancer.[148]

An umbrella review of 96 meta-analyses suggests that tea consumption shows greater benefits than harm to health.[149] Two to three cups of tea daily reduce the risks of type 2 diabetes, total mortality, cardiac death, heart disease, and stroke.

Does adding milk reduce the antioxidant activity of tea? Yes, but not significantly. If you want to squeeze every cup's maximum possible health benefit, ditch the milk. If you enjoy your tea with milk, you may continue providing you keep track of the type of milk, the number of cups per day, and the sugar or sweetener added. However, a squeeze of lemon enhances white tea's antioxidant content due to the pH change.[150]

Amla

Amla, the Indian gooseberry, is a superfood or should I say, Superfruit, as it's the single most antioxidant-packed fruit in nature. Amla is high in soluble and insoluble fibre, vitamin C, chromium, and chlorogenic acid.

Several research studies have evidenced the use of this powerful fruit for benefits on blood glucose, blood pressure, cholesterol, and improving immunity.[151] A study in 2011 showed that when people with diabetes were fed one, two, and three grams of amla powder every day for 21 days, they improved their fasting and post-meal blood glucose and lipid profile.[152]

The fruit is excessively sour, so eating it raw could depend on your palate. However, you can incorporate it in your salads, drinks, curries, sauces, or fresh juices.

Bright Fruits and Vegetables

Polyphenols are micronutrients found in the bright colors of fruits and vegetables and have an incredibly positive effect on inflammation. For example, fruits like berries; leafy greens like spinach and kale; and vegetables like tomatoes and beets. While eggplants have nice, dark skin, the flesh is white, so it isn't a high polyphenol choice.

Spinach, collards, and kale are dark green leafy vegetables packed with vitamins and minerals, such as vitamins A, C, E, and K; iron; calcium; and potassium. These powerhouse foods are low in calories and carbohydrates, too. Try adding dark leafy vegetables to salads, soups, and stews.

Dark Chocolate

Eat a little dark chocolate more often to increase your intake of polyphenols and prebiotics. Remember to practice mindful eating when putting that piece of the best dark chocolate (at least 70% cacao) in your mouth. Let it sit on or under your tongue and roll it gently until it slowly dissolves in your mouth. Not only will you enjoy the chocolate, but it also stimulates the production of endorphins (happy mood hormones) that are 200 times more powerful than morphine in how they stimulate the feel-good sensors in your brain.

If you have eaten 1 square of chocolate and let it melt in your mouth for a good 2 minutes, you will likely feel satisfied. If you wish to have another square, remember the mindful eating practice. This way, you can have dark chocolate and not spike your blood glucose or gain weight.

Glucose-lowering foods

Plant foods are abundant in bioactive functional compounds that offer a wide array of health benefits. Throughout history, specific food adjuncts have been recognized for their therapeutic potential in disease management, thanks to their beneficial phytonutrients like phenolics, flavonoids, alkaloids, polyphenols, glycosides, terpenoids, and polysaccharides. Moreover, recent research has shed light on the role of certain foods in controlling plasma glucose levels, further highlighting their potential in promoting overall well-being.[153]

Fenugreek

Fenugreek is an aromatic plant with many uses, both culinary (a key ingredient in curries and other Indian recipes) and medicinal. Fenugreek seeds are high in soluble fibre that helps lower blood sugar by slowing down digestion and the absorption of carbohydrates. This suggests they may be effective in treating people with diabetes.

Multiple studies have been carried out to investigate the potential antidiabetic benefits of fenugreek.[154] A randomised controlled trial showed that incorporating 15 grams of powdered fenugreek seed into a meal eaten by people with type 2 diabetes reduced the rise in post-meal blood glucose.[155] At the same time, a separate study found that taking 2.5 grams of fenugreek twice a day for 3 months lowered blood glucose levels in people with fairly controlled type 2 diabetes.[156]

Results from a meta-analysis of clinical trials support the beneficial effects of fenugreek seeds on glycaemic control in people with diabetes. Nevertheless, significant effects on fasting and 2-hour glucose were only found in studies that administered medium or high doses of fenugreek (5-25 grams/day).[157]

Extra Virgin Olive Oil

Extra virgin olive oil is the main source of dietary fat in the Mediterranean diet. It has a high content of monounsaturated fatty acids (MUFA) and phenolic compounds like tyrosol, secoiridoids, and lignans. Compared with refined olive oil, extra virgin olive oil contains a fourfold (232 vs. 62 mg/kg) amount of phenolic compounds.[158] Studies show that adding extra virgin olive oil to a high-glycemic index meal helps reduce the body's glycemic response.[159]

A 2017 meta-analysis found that people consuming the most olive oil had, on average, a 16% reduced risk of developing type 2 diabetes and significant reductions in fasting blood sugar and HbA1c levels. Finally, compounds in extra virgin olive oil have been shown to reduce inflammation and oxidative stress—two factors that can contribute to diabetes and diabetes complications.[160]

Remember that this is an oil, and it contributes the same 9 kcal per gram as any other oil. Use olive oil as a replacement for other oils not as an addition.

Cinnamon

Cinnamon is made from the dried bark of Cinnamomum trees and is a commonly used spice added to sweet and savory dishes worldwide. Various beneficial effects of cinnamon, such as antimicrobial, anti-inflammatory, antioxidant, antifungal, and antidiabetic properties, have been reported.[161, 162]

The tolerable daily intake of cinnamon has been determined to be 0.1 mg per kg/day to ensure safe use.[163, 164] For example, if you weigh 70 kg, you could limit your intake to below 7 grams daily. A teaspoon (2-4 grams) of powder per day is suggested by some experts. Cinnamon has been used safely in some studies between 1 gram and 6 grams, but high doses may be toxic. [165, 166]

From a clinical viewpoint, it's often used in diabetes treatment because of its hypoglycaemic and lipid-lowering potential. It has also been found to be useful in reducing glycated haemoglobin (HbA1c) and fasting blood glucose levels in patients with type 2 diabetes.[167]

2. Tweak with Continuous Glucose Monitoring

Your goal is almost within reach. Congratulations. To make these changes successful permanently, you need to adapt them to your daily lifestyle choices and observe how they affect your blood glucose levels throughout the day by using continuous glucose monitoring (CGM).

CGM has recently become an increasingly available choice for self-monitoring glucose levels over an extended period, and it can be highly effective, too. Even though there are several types of CGM devices, they all function in the same way.

A small sensor is inserted just under the skin, usually on the abdomen or the back of the upper arms. This sensor measures interstitial glucose (glucose that has left the blood and has moved into the tissues) and can be worn for up to 14 days.

It takes glucose readings as frequently as every 5 minutes that you can then see on your smartphone or on a wireless handheld device specifically designed for CGM. Some CGM devices include features like a virtual notepad or an accompanying app for tracking your meals or an alarm if your blood sugar levels are too high or too low.

Even if you have a good handle on your diabetes management, you still may want to consider using a CGM for the convenience and elimination of finger pricks. This could help you and your healthcare providers in understanding the pattern and identifying the red flags in your glucose control pattern in a 24-hour cycle.

In Chapters 2 and 4, you learned that HbA1c reflects the average glucose level over the past 60-90 days, but it won't tell you the number or levels of low and high glucose. Pre and post-meal glucose finger pricks give you information about meal choices and the action of any medication on the meals. However, the time spent between meals and during sleep goes unrecorded. Hence the complete view that a CGM device gives throughout the 24 hours makes it easy to identify any specific area of concern and deal with it effectively.

The user must scan the sensor with a smartphone (app) or a reader to see the glucose reading. Updated readings are available every 1 minute, if scanned. The sensor must be scanned at least once every 8 hours to capture all the data to review in graphs later. Set your target glucose reading between 70 and 180 mg/dl (3.9 to 10 mmol/l) and monitor it throughout the day.

The added advantage of this is that a CGM alerts the user that a glucose level is out of target.

When looking to understand the data consider these points:

- Individual daily profiles—check the variation in glucose throughout the 24 hours and identify the red flags.
- Note the changes in late night, midnight, early morning, fasting, pre-meal, and post-meal phases.
- Look at the impact of other factors, such as exercise, stress, work patterns, and sleep patterns.
- Keep trying variations in meal patterns, portions, proportion, and food items and check the fluctuations and identify the food items or meals that increase your blood glucose beyond the target.

3. Lapse, Relapse, Improvise, and Repeat

Even with a well-thought-out plan and the best intentions, you may face challenges now and then. How you respond to these obstacles can be the difference between success and failure. Don't beat yourself up for a lapse, just get right back on track. It's not what you do once that determines your health but what you do consistently.

Relapse is more serious. After several lapses have occurred in a short period, you are at risk of losing your new healthy habits and falling back into the way things were. During a relapse, you may panic and feel like it's all been a waste of time and you have 'ruined' it.

Calm down, take a deep breath, and get things in context. In most cases, a lapse happens when your routine is shifted for some reason. These tips will help you identify what has happened and why, and get back on track so that the lapses don't become relapses:

Be Mindful of Your Thoughts and Feelings

When you feel you are slipping away from your new habits, stop, take a breath, and observe. Recognise what's happening, make room for accepting what has happened, investigate why it's happening without judging, and find ways of doing it differently.

For example, you visit a restaurant you haven't been to before and you choose the 'wrong' meal. That's OK. Now you know you need to investigate the menu more before you go back next time. Spot the problem area and enlist objective possible solutions. (For more solutions, see Chapter 5).

Seek Support

Talk to family, friends, or a professional counsellor. Involving significant others in your decisions and activities helps cement the changes.

Avoid Boredom

If boredom is one of your triggers leading to emotional eating, then it will be important to keep active. Taking up a new hobby or exercise routine will help avoid the trigger of 'boredom eating.'

Learn Compensation Skills

There's no doubt that participating in social situations with family, friends, and coworkers can be one of the most difficult aspects of adhering to the 5C program. The external social environment can significantly impact your decisions and ability to stick to the program. Knowing this, create a game plan that suits you the best.

For example, have a small high-protein meal before your planned event. This will keep you full for a long time and avoid emotional decisions made at a party. If you know you are likely to exceed your calorie allowance at the party then compensate in the meals before and/or after.

This works with my patients as they can still enjoy the party without feeling guilty or without depriving themselves at the party. The other way to compensate is by increasing your activity, like walking or adding extra minutes in your gym session.

What If You Relapse?

Although relapses are disappointing, they can still teach you a lot about your strengths and weaknesses. If you see them as a normal part of life and a learning opportunity rather than the end of your journey. Just get back on the wagon. Reverting to old habits and behaviours doesn't mean you should lose hope or that you have failed. It just means you need to recharge your motivation and recommit to your journey to be healthy and happy.

Take Home Messages:

1. Journaling is a powerful tool for self-improvement, helping you identify patterns, become more mindful, and make decisions aligned with your goals.
2. Examine your grocery list, differentiate between real food and ultra-processed foods.
3. One simple way to promote healthy eating is to carefully consider the proportion and portion of each food group on your plate.
4. Carbohydrate-rich food groups include grains, fruits, milk and yoghurt, beans/legumes, and starchy vegetables.
5. Mediterranean diets, which emphasize plant-based and minimally processed foods, have consistently shown to improve glycaemic control, cardiovascular health, weight loss, and reducing chronic disease risk.
6. Maintaining optimal blood glucose control requires vigilance over your fasting, pre-meal, and post-meal glucose concentrations. Stay mindful of these levels and make necessary adjustments to ensure the best results.

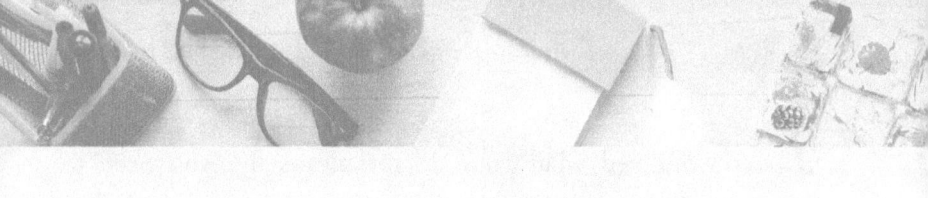

CHAPTER 8

THE 4ᵀᴴ C - COUNT ON ACTIVE MOVEMENT, SOUND SLEEP, AND RELAXATION

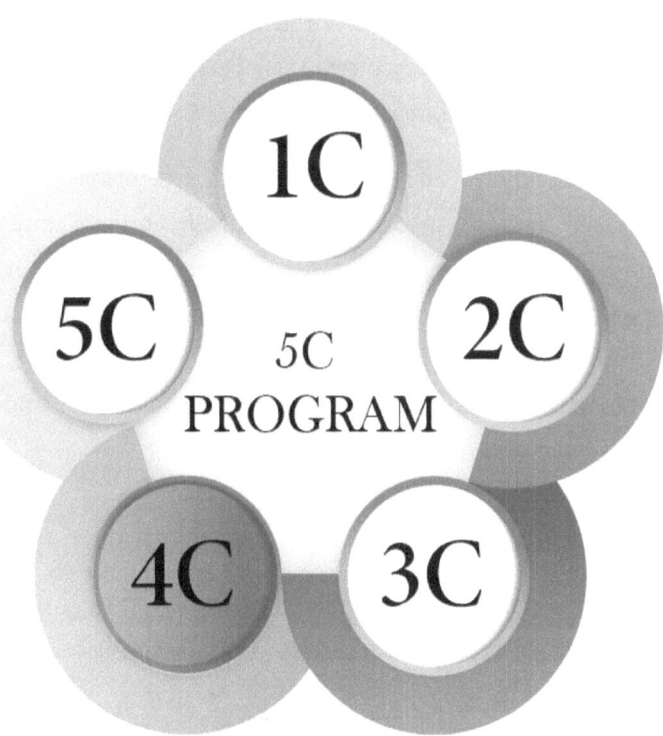

*E*ver wondered what your doctor means by "you need to change your lifestyle?" It's a gentle reminder that if you don't start prioritizing healthy eating, exercise, sleep, and stress reduction, you might find yourself making frequent visits to their office for more tests and medications. A lifestyle change is like a deposit in the bank of health; it takes a while to accrue, but the dividends will pay off in the long run. The goal of lifestyle changes is not just better blood sugar, but better health and a better quality of life.

But let's face it, we all wish for a magic pill that could solve all our health issues in an instant! What if I told you that such magic pills exist that can reduce bad cholesterol, make your bones and muscles stronger, improve your immunity, relieve your stress, help you think clearly, improve your personal relationships, and above all, keep your blood glucose under control?

The catch is, there's one condition: you need to make a promise to yourself to create space for it in your life and integrate it into your daily routine. Getting active, prioritizing sufficient sleep, and practicing relaxation techniques are the magic pills that form the foundation of the 4th C in this program. So, are you ready to embrace these transformative habits and unlock the true potential of a healthier and happier life?

Active Movement

Bob Butler, the founding director of the National Institute on Ageing once declared, "If exercise could be packaged in a pill, it would be the single most widely prescribed and beneficial medicine in the nation." Now, almost 50 years later, scientists have added strength to this statement with several research studies.[168]

Other than dietary changes, the most powerful defense tool for people living with diabetes or people trying to prevent the development of diabetes and other chronic diseases is movement. I prefer the word movement to 'exercise.'

When you think about the word "exercise," the image created in your mind is often not pleasant; it sounds like something that is tiring, painful, stressful, annoying – an effort! And this closes the process before it opens, and you may think:

- Exercise is not for me.
- I don't have the time for this hard work.
- Even if I start, I won't be able to continue.

You know, of course, that physical activity is helpful for your physical and mental health. Research has shown that physical inactivity is closely correlated to heart disease, diabetes, and certain cancers (breast and colon). A study by Lee et al. in Lancet showed that physical inactivity causes 6% of coronary heart disease and 7% of type 2 diabetes.[169]

Research studies have suggested that half a million deaths would be prevented if people added 10 percent more physical activity to their daily lives. Every 10 minutes of active movement knocks off a certain degree of risk of diseases and death.[170] Needless to say, the benefits of physical movement are nothing less than a magic pill.

What to Do Before You Start?

As quoted by Benjamin Franklin, "By failing to prepare, you are preparing to fail."

To avoid failure, preparation is the key, and you may need to condition yourself before changing your behaviour. (Refer to 1C in Chapter 5.)

First, think about the word exercise and note what images you see in your mind—this is your present perception of exercise. If you have seen a tiring, boring gym session, walking alone, or pushing a bicycle and feeling exhausted, you need to work on these negative associations first.

When we are not sleeping, we should be engaged in some form of physical movement. Our metabolism and physiology have evolved so that our bodies can move around, perform activities, and use our muscles for our well-being. Any form of movement that results in burning energy is a form of physical activity.

Let's start by replacing the term exercise with "active movement." Movement is normal, natural and not 'forced' as exercise can appear to be. Movement should be your choice and preference. There's no need to go to a gym if that fills you with dread!

Active movement is about finding something that you love to do and that causes you to break a sweat. Find a window of time and figure out how to do those things you love. And it can be anything from household chores, gardening, walking your dog, chasing a ball around with your children, mindful walking with music or listening to your favourite book or religious sermons, or dancing to your favourite number and breaking a sweat.

Now, whenever you want to engage in your choice of 'active movement' I encourage you to swap thinking about how you might feel about it BEFORE (not looking forward to it) to how you will feel AFTER—which could be feeling proud of yourself, happy or energetic.

Remember: the type of movement doesn't matter, but to make it even more effective, you should add to it over time. For example, make the walk longer, or faster, or both! Buy some wrist or ankle weights and wear them while dancing. Rather than trying to carry everything upstairs at once when doing housework, take one thing at a time and make the stair climbing part of the routine. Park the car further away from the shops and walk further each week.

How Active Movement Improves Your Blood Glucose?

Taking care of your body is similar to doing regular maintenance on your car. Just as doing oil changes and tune-ups regularly will keep your car running better and for longer, exercising regularly will help keep your body functioning at its finest. Besides maintaining your overall health, physical activity also helps control your glucose levels to reduce your risk of illness.

One of the reasons why physical activity reduces blood glucose levels is that it increases muscle mass and reduces body fat percentage. This improves insulin sensitivity, resulting in better blood glucose control. Reduced blood pressure and blood lipids are also added benefits.

Let's look at why and how active physical movement influences your blood glucose on a short-term and long-term basis.

Exercise and Mitochondrial Function

The energy from carbohydrates, fats and proteins source is burned in tiny furnaces called mitochondria in the cells to release high-energy compounds called Adenosine Triphosphate (ATP). When you engage in physical movement, these mitochondria increase the rate of ATP production by as much as 100 times—increasing your energy-burning capacity. The results of a large body of human physiological studies suggest that insulin resistance is closely linked to and may cause reduced mitochondrial function, and physical exercise may be able to mitigate it.[171]

Mitochondria are also involved in the release of insulin from pancreatic beta cells. So we can see that mitochondrial dysfunction is a defect that leads to type 2 diabetes by affecting the release of insulin and insulin resistance.[172]

Furthermore, when you work at high intensity, your body, particularly your muscles, needs an extra supply of energy created by the mitochondria. The most effective way to produce mitochondria in muscles is through active movement.

Therefore, increasing active movement can indirectly improve mitochondrial function and improve insulin sensitivity.[173]

Exercises Improve Glucose Transporter Channels

If you could recall from Chapter 2, insulin opens the doors to the liver and muscle cells for glucose, and in diabetics, this doesn't work properly. When we go down to the cellular level, these glucose transporters (doors) are called GLUT4.

The good news is that physical exercise can open these doors, and glucose enters the cell without needing insulin. When you exercise, your body naturally lowers the glucose levels because it flows into the cell without the need for insulin or needs much lesser insulin than needed otherwise, and your body can use less insulin over time.[174]

Now, another thing that exercise does is it up-regulates the genes that add more GLUT4 receptors. So, as you exercise over time, you are using the GLUT4 receptors that you have and producing more of them. Eventually, your insulin requirements come down through just the regular addition of exercise.

Exercise and Happy Hormones

Exercise does a lot of other wonderful things for the body. It stimulates the release of endorphins and epinephrine in the brain and adrenaline. Research has shown that when people exercise, and their mood is better, they make better choices with their food after exercising rather than when they are physically inactive.[175]

I think that's often missed when we talk about exercise because we talked about the other benefits like calorie burning, increased lung capacity and muscle building. But that mood component is critically important, especially in our culture of bad choices around food.

How to Get Started?

Before you start a new exercise program, consult with your doctor to check your heart is up to it. Are you on any medications that make you vulnerable to hypo or hyperglycemia (low or high blood glucose)? Do you have any concerns with your feet (neuropathy) or eyes (retinopathy) that can worsen with exercise? Your healthcare team can help you to adjust your exercise plan based on your medications and contraindications.

Rest assured, there is always a way to start exercising. Walking is the safest way to start, and you can start small and build on it.

Do All Exercises Have the Same Effect on Your Body?

The simple answer to this is NO! Different kinds of exercises provide very different benefits. Hence, exercise recommendations are not based solely on time and duration, but also on exercise type.

Types of Exercises

a. Aerobic exercise (Cardiovascular): This is an activity in which large muscles are moved rhythmically for a sustained period. You can begin from as little as 5 minutes to more than an hour. This exercise improves cardiovascular fitness and reduces blood glucose and triglyceride levels (fat cells in the blood). Examples include brisk walking, cycling, dancing, playing, swimming, and using a treadmill or elliptical trainer, and many other sports.

b. Strength training (Resistance training): The purpose of these exercises is to improve strength by building a muscle or muscle group. Consequently, these exercises result in:
   i. Increase of basal metabolic rate (rate of burning calories)
   ii. Reduced fatigue
   iii. Improved sleep, muscle strength, and bone density

In people with diabetes, these exercises improve health by reducing body fat, lipid profile, and insulin resistance.

Examples are climbing stairs, using a treadmill with an incline, using an exercise bike with resistance, weight training, push-ups, sit-ups, squats, and working with resistance bands, just to name a few.

c. Flexibility (stretching): Every joint in your body needs a specific set of exercises to maintain its range of motion and these exercises help in maintaining the flexibility and overall fitness of your muscles. For example, stretching exercises, such as Yoga, Pilates, and Tai Chi.

d. Balance: Balancing exercises work your core muscles, lower back, and legs. Lower-body strength-training exercises can also help improve your balance.

How Long and How Often to Exercise?

Before you plan your exercise prescription, assess yourself for your current daily activity level, intensity, and fitness. It's like a doctor prescribing medicine; before they can do so, they must assess the patient's current health status. Similarly, you should assess yourself before you plan your exercise prescription to know what level of intensity and fitness you are capable of.

Assess Your Baseline Activity Level into One of the Four Categories

1. Inactive: No active physical movement beyond basic daily chores
2. Low: Beyond basic daily chores but fewer than 150 minutes per week
3. Medium: Beyond basic daily chores, additional 150-300 minutes per week
4. High: Beyond basic daily chores, more than 300 minutes per week

Assess the Intensity of the Exercise by the "Talk Test"

1. Low intensity: Activity where you can talk or sing while exercising.
2. Moderate intensity: when talking is comfortable, but singing becomes difficult.
3. Vigorous intensity: neither singing nor prolonged talking is possible.

Assess Your Fitness

Fitness is the capability to perform daily tasks with energy and alertness and without undue fatigue. Fitness tests are a great way to check your fitness level when beginning a new workout routine. Tests vary; for instance, a 6-minute treadmill test, a plank test, a pushup or sit-up test, and a sit and reach test. You may choose the test that is most relevant for you.

By having a baseline, you can track your progress. If you can only walk on a treadmill for 5 minutes before becoming out of breath when you start and 3 weeks later, you can walk for 20 minutes—that is progress. Write your fitness test results in your journal or record them in your favourite fitness app to better track your progress.

Rule of Thumb for How Long and How Often to Exercise

If you have a green signal from your physician and are just beginning or resuming exercise, start slowly with maybe 5–10 minutes based on your fitness level. Then, gradually build up over time, the duration, intensity, and type of active movement. The American Diabetic Association and Heart Association recommends at least 150 minutes (2 ½ hours) of moderate-intensity activity besides daily household chores every week. 5–10 minutes of warm-up and cool-down will reduce your chances of injuries and soreness.[176]

The Magic Number: 150

It takes 150 minutes every week to keep your blood glucose in check. It can seem daunting to dedicate that much time to exercise if you are busy, dislike working out, or have diabetes-related complications that make active movement difficult. You don't need to worry: 150 minutes of exercise will be easier than you think!

These 150 minutes can be spread based on the following factors:

- Fitness level
- Goals
- Motivation

Make it 30 minutes 5 times/week or 25 minutes 6 times. The key is to keep pushing yourself to reach up to 300 minutes/week of moderate-intensity activity.

Active Movement-Everyday

Throughout the day, be mindful of how much time you spend moving and how much sitting. Simple behaviours of sitting for a prolonged time in front of a screen, desk, etc., have damaging effects on heart health. Prolonged sitting should be interrupted every 30 minutes for blood glucose benefit. So, ensure you get up and move at least for 5 minutes every 20-30 minutes of sitting for better blood glucose. Walking for 15 minutes after a meal also brings down your blood glucose. Make these small activities for a compound effect on overall blood glucose control.

You can make these 150 minutes even better by adding strength training exercises twice a week and flexibility and balance exercises twice a week.

Figure 8.1 Activity and exercise pyramid

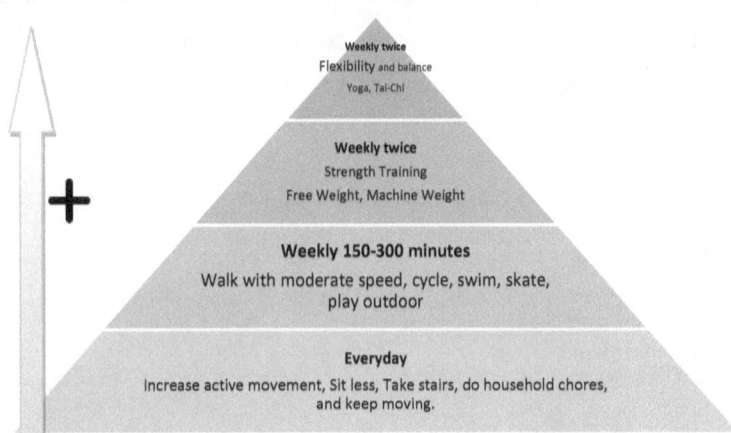

Active Movement and Insulin Action

Aside from the other benefits of movement on overall health, exercise is crucial for lowering blood glucose levels. Since diabetes is caused by inefficient insulin metabolism, it is important to remember that with regular active movement, the amount of insulin your body requires to maintain blood glucose decreases. In other words, exercise is like an additional medication for people with type 2 diabetes. Moreover, research studies on people with diabetes taking injectable insulin have shown that their need for external insulin was reduced significantly when the patients included daily active movement in their routine.[177, 178]

The type, duration, and intensity with which you exercise can dramatically affect blood glucose for the next 24 to 48 hours. All forms of exercise deplete glucose and fatty acids that are the stored fuel (glycogen and triglyceride) in the liver, muscles, and adipose tissues, as well as inhibiting glucose production from the liver.

Glucose is preferably used for short-duration, higher-intensity aerobic exercises like speed walking, running, and high-intensity interval training (HIIT). As a result of HIIT, post-meal glucose spikes are reduced, and insulin sensitivity is increased in skeletal muscle without the need for insulin. It is like priming a pump; by doing HIIT, your body is better able to use the nutrients that it is taking in and lessen the negative consequences of consuming these nutrients. Long-term interval training reduces HbA1c levels in people with a high risk of diabetes and those diagnosed with type 2 diabetes.[179]

But you don't have to go for high intensity if this doesn't suit you or your fitness is not yet at that level.

Pilates is a form of low-impact exercise that aims to strengthen muscles while improving postural alignment and flexibility and a review of 15 clinical trials have concluded that this form of exercise could improve post-meal blood glucose, fasting blood glucose, HbA1c, Triglycerides, total cholesterol, and LDL-Cholesterol for diabetic patients, which could be influenced by its duration and intensity.[180]

Remember to keep moving consciously and build up your schedule based on the exercise build-up pyramid to get the maximum benefit for your blood glucose and heart health.

How can you manage your blood glucose before, during, and after exercises?

Exercise usually makes your blood glucose level go down. Ensure that you read this section carefully for safe, optimum blood glucose if you relate to the following health situation.

- Have poorly controlled glucose.
- Are on insulin.
- Are at risk of ketones.
- Have been diagnosed with complications of diabetes.

Before Exercise

Check your blood glucose before you start exercising. The target range for blood glucose before exercise should ideally be between 90 and 250 mg/dL (5.0 and 13.9 mmol/L). However, you need to figure out your optimum pre-workout blood glucose range by experimenting a few times to check blood sugar before, during, and after exercises and be mindful of hypoglycaemia and hyperglycaemia.

If you are on oral medications alone:

Blood glucose decreases during and after exercise for individuals with type 2 diabetes; however, this does not usually result in hypoglycaemia unless the individual is taking insulin or sulphonylureas.

Start your exercise within a safe limit of 100 and 250 mg/dL and monitor for a few days for post-exercise. If your blood glucose levels are within the recommended target range after the exercise session, you may continue. If your glucose is dropping rapidly or is below 100mg/dl, you may consume one portion of a carbohydrate snack before you start your exercise session and raise the lower limit of your safe limit to 120-250mg/dl for the next exercise session and check again. If you see a rapid increase in blood glucose while and after exercising, you should lower the upper limit of your safe limit to 100-200mg/dL.

If you Inject insulin:

If you are diagnosed with type 1 diabetes mellitus, slightly elevate your blood glucose before the exercise session to prevent unwarranted hypo's. You could start with a safe range of 150-250 mg/dl (8.3–13.9 mmol/L) and adjust as you get familiar with how your body responds to the exercise type, duration, and intensity.[181]

- If the blood glucose is lower than the safe limit, consume a carbohydrate snack (approx. 15-20 gm) before you start. For instance, an apple, 1 cup yoghurt, one piece of toast or half a banana and have a safe pre-exercise glucose limit.
- If the blood glucose is between 250 to 350 mg/dl (13.9–19.4 mmol/L), test for ketones (chemicals that the body creates when it breaks down fat to use for energy when it doesn't have enough insulin) and continue with low-intensity exercise. Also, avoid moderate to high-intensity activities or preferably wait until the levels reach the safe limit.

The American Diabetes Association (ADA) recommends 10-15 gm of carbohydrates before a low- to moderate-intensity aerobic activity lasting 30-60 min (in fasting or 3- 4 hours after meals state).

As an alternative or a complement to carbohydrate intake, consider reductions in your insulin dose for exercise-induced hypoglycemia prevention; lowering insulin levels adequately during activity may reduce or eliminate the need for carbohydrate intake. The ADA recommends a 50% reduction in pre-exercise meal insulin bolus reduction for activity started within 90 min after insulin administration.[182] It is advisable to discuss this with your doctor!

Proper documentation for two weeks is key to understanding your safe pre-exercise blood glucose range and how to adjust carbohydrate and/or insulin dosage.

What and when to eat before exercise

Depending on your pre-exercise blood glucose, intensity, and duration of exercise, you may choose healthy carbohydrate-rich snacks like fruits, starchy vegetables, whole grains or beans. Fruits are the best choice as they move faster through your digestive system and raise your blood glucose more quickly than whole grains, beans, and vegetables do. Try to keep away from ultra-processed carbohydrate-based snacks like cookies, biscuits, or soda. For prolonged activity, you may need to eat a small carbohydrate snack before, during, or after exercise.

When do I need to snack before an exercise session?

1. If your blood glucose level is less than 100 mg/dl before exercise
2. If your blood glucose level is between 100-150mg/dl before exercise AND you will exercise for more than 1 hour
3. If your blood glucose level usually falls below 100mg/dl during exercise
4. If your blood glucose level is below 100mg/dl after exercise

During Exercise

Most of the time, working out causes blood glucose to dip. But some people notice a rise in blood glucose levels during or after a particular exercise. Fear not! There are steps you can take to avoid this. Some workouts, such as heavy weightlifting, sprints, and competitive sports, cause you to produce stress hormones (such as adrenaline). Adrenaline raises blood glucose levels by stimulating your liver to release glucose.

Sometimes, the food you eat before or during a workout may also increase glucose. Eating too many carbohydrates before exercising or indulging in sugar-loaded energy drinks while exercising can push your blood glucose levels up during and after exercises. Exercising early in the morning (between 4:00 AM to 8:00 AM) signals the liver to boost the production of glucose due to the "dawn phenomenon" (an early-morning rise in blood sugar due to the release of hormones like cortisol and growth hormone); this, in turn, provides energy that helps you wake up.

How to keep blood glucose from rising during and after workouts

 i. Shift to moderate-intensity aerobic workouts or circuit weight training with light weights and high repetitions.
 ii. Practice relaxation techniques such as paced breathing, visualisation, or meditation before and during your workout to minimize the adrenaline effect.
 iii. Consider moving your workout to later in the day if you usually exercise in the early mornings. To prevent the effects of the dawn phenomenon on blood glucose, the same workout done later in the day is less likely to result in a rise.
 iv. Talk with your doctor/diabetes educator if you are on multiple daily dose injections of insulin or an insulin pump for adjusting your doses based on the time, duration, and intensity of your workout.
 v. Avoid eating excessive amounts of carbohydrates before and during your workouts. Try to be watchful of sports drinks loaded with sugar.

However, if you exercise high intensity, monitor your blood glucose closely throughout the exercise session. Continuous glucose monitoring devices will be a great advantage in making informed decisions in these situations.

While learning how your body responds to exercises, keep the blood glucose throughout the session in a safe range of 120-150 mg/dl and be mindful of how you are feeling.

After Exercise

Exercise depletes glucose and fatty acids from your blood into exercising muscle so that the muscle can burn them for energy. Sounds similar to what insulin does, right? Insulin also transports glucose and fatty acids from the blood into the liver, muscles, and adipose tissues.

Because of this, active physical movement acts as a proxy for insulin, and it remains in your body for 24 to 48 hours, depending on the type, duration, and intensity of the activity. What better deal can you ask for?

What to eat after exercise?

Getting the right nutrients after exercise can help stabilise your blood glucose and rebuild your muscle proteins and glycogen stores. If you're trying to lose weight and your workouts are lower in intensity (like walking, cycling, yoga, swimming for less than an hour), you likely do not need an intentional "post-workout meal." Instead, strive to eat mostly your regular healthy meals throughout the day to support your calorie needs.

However, if you are indulging in a high-intensity activity session like HIIT, competitive sports (tennis, soccer, skiing etc.), or any intense exercise for more than an hour, eating a meal high in protein and carbohydrates after the session is important.

To replenish your muscles' stored glucose (glycogen) and provide amino acids (protein building blocks) to rebuild the muscle tissue. Intense training requires proper fuel. Eating every three to four hours throughout the day and eating post-workout is important to support your body.

If you inject insulin:

Let's suppose you had a high-intensity interval training session at the gym in the evening, and your blood sugars have been good all day. Crawling into bed and falling asleep feels glorious. Best day ever! In the middle of the night, you dream of nightmares and feel so exhausted that you shake and sweat uncontrollably. You wake up to low blood glucose. You could think, 'Why did this happen? My sugars were good all day!'

Night-time hypoglycaemia after exercise is common for people with type 1 diabetes. One of the causes of late-onset hypoglycaemia is that the body is more sensitive to insulin after exercise, and this effect can last for 24 to 48 hours. The more intense and prolonged the activity, the longer and greater the insulin sensitivity. Muscles must replenish their energy stores (glycogen) following long-duration exercise. Hence, hypoglycemia may result if sufficient carbohydrate is not consumed in the hours following exercise.

If you take mealtime insulin or other medications that can cause low blood sugars, you'll need to plan the timing of your meals and your exercise more carefully. A high-intensity exercise session within 3 hours of your regular meal with regular insulin can cause low blood glucose. This is because exercise acts as a proxy/substitute for insulin action. This means you'd need less insulin to manage your goal blood sugar levels after that meal.

If an insufficient amount of carbohydrates is consumed after exercise, the risk of late-onset, post-exercise hypoglycemia may be increased. Have a snack that is a combination of slow-releasing carbohydrates and proteins, for example, fruit yoghurt or plain yoghurt, milk, nuts with plant-based milk, an egg sandwich or peanut butter with whole-grain toast.

Reduce the amount of insulin you take for that meal depending on the intensity and duration of your workout (you may start with a 50% reduced dose) and keep a record for a week to adjust accordingly. If you are on an insulin pump, consult your healthcare provider to determine how and if you should adjust insulin doses before and after exercise.

Both decreasing insulin doses and increasing carbohydrate intake can help minimise the chance of having delayed-onset hypoglycemia. Remember, there will be some trial and error. Keep good records and analyse them with the help of your healthcare team. Don't let your experience or fear of low blood glucose prevent you from being active.

Sleep and Blood Glucose

If you are a shift worker who goes to work after dinner and returns before sunrise, you know how it feels to be living against a primitive, primordial drive to sleep at night and stay awake during the day. But even if you're not, I'm sure you can remember a time when you pulled an all-nighter at university or work, stayed up late finishing that assignment, traveled across time zones, or stayed awake for your sick child.

That one night of inadequate sleep left you tired, moody, nauseated, and forgetful. If one or two days of poor sleep could impact your body and brain, then the chronic effect of inadequate sleep could wreck your physical and mental health.

Humans are endowed with a circadian clock—an internally driven 24-hour rhythm that resets every day by the sun's light/dark cycle. Our daily rhythms guide our entire sense of health. Circadian rhythms optimise biological functions. Every function in the body has a specific time because the body cannot accomplish all its needs to do at once.

In the morning, being in good health means waking up feeling rested and refreshed from having a good night's sleep. In the evening, good health means winding down, feeling tired, and falling into deep sleep without much effort. Sleep is not a dormant mode where the brain shuts down. On the contrary, the brain is very active while we sleep, consolidating memories from the information. The pineal gland releases melatonin—a sleep hormone—when it gets dark.

The human body is like a well-oiled machine when everything happens when and as it should. When you disrupt the schedule, it creates havoc. For instance, energy-sensing pathway cells, hunger, and satiety (fullness) are controlled by a circadian rhythm, where you feel hungry during the day and do not feel too hungry at night. This is not by chance.

Every cell in every organ has a mechanism that makes the cell hungry for energy and opens its doors for nutrients during the day. When the cells have enough energy, they tend to close the doors at night.[183]

Poor Circadian Rhythms Are Linked to Type 2 Diabetes.

We understood earlier that type 2 diabetes is caused by insulin resistance and beta cell dysfunction. However, there is now mounting evidence that poor sleep behaviour disrupting the circadian rhythm can lead to diabetes. For instance, even partial sleep deprivation over one night increases insulin resistance, which can increase blood sugar levels.[184] You can imagine prolonged sleep deprivation can push you into the consequences of insulin resistance, which are type 2 diabetes, cardiovascular diseases, and obesity, to name a few.

Scientists have reported, based on several studies, that glucose metabolism in people with type 2 diabetes shows an increase in insulin resistance and liver glucose production across the night in anticipation of awakening in the morning, contributing to high fasting blood glucose. As mentioned, this is the well-known, 'Dawn phenomenon'.[185]

During the night, the pancreas's circadian cycle slows insulin release. In addition, the circadian cycle of the brain produces melatonin at night, which acts on the pancreas to further lessen the release of insulin. Now that the insulin levels are lower at night, the glucose levels peak quickly. As a result, if you sleep late and snack at night when the pancreas is half asleep, you will have dangerously high glucose levels, and chronic hyperglycaemia is known to speed up diabetic complications of the eyes, kidneys, nerves, and heart.

When maintaining good glucose control, we must focus not only on diet and medication but also focus on creating optimum sleep behaviour.

How Much is Too Much or Too Little?

The magic number for metabolically optimised sleep appears to be between **seven to eight hours** per night. Less than seven and the risk of diabetes increases sharply for every hour lost. Above eight hours, the risk also increases.

What Causes Sleep Disturbances?

Inadequate Sleep: This is a voluntary restriction of sleep time (you do not get an adequate 7-9 hours of sleep/day). This is a behaviour-induced disorder. Our behaviour governs our sleeping routines, so it is essential to dig deeper into the reason for this behaviour and try to change it a little at a time to better control glucose levels. Is it that your workload has meant that you have sacrificed sleep? Or are you of the opinion (as some workaholics believe) that sleep is a waste of time?

Insomnia: With insomnia, you may have trouble falling asleep, staying asleep, getting back to sleep after waking or getting good quality sleep. This happens even if you have the time and the right environment to sleep well. Insomnia can get in the way of your daily activities and may make you feel sleepy during the day.

Obstructive Sleep Apnea: This is a common and serious sleep disorder that causes you to stop breathing during sleep. The block in airflow is usually caused by the collapse of the soft tissues in the back of the throat and tongue during sleep. When this happens, you may snore loudly or make choking noises as you try to breathe. Your brain and body become oxygen-deprived, and you may wake up. Breathing pauses can last from a few seconds to minutes.

Sleep apnea can make you wake up in the morning feeling tired or un-refreshed even though you have had a full night of sleep. Besides keeping you from feeling rested, it can produce insulin resistance too.

Unfortunately, most people are unaware that they have sleep apnea. Fortunately, some treatments can be effective. Consult your physician to refer you to a sleep clinic.

Tips and Tricks to Improve Sleep Hygiene

Getting a good night's sleep is easier said than done. However, lifestyle changes can significantly improve your sleep. Too often, suggestions for sleep improvement require sweeping life changes that just aren't realistic for most people. There is no one-size fits all recommendation; it needs to be tailored based on your needs, priorities, resources, commitments, and goals[186] but the following can help.

During the Day Time

1. Expose yourself to bright daylight, preferably outdoors.

Light, especially natural light is the key driver of your circadian rhythm, which regulates sleep-wake patterns. Exposure to morning and early afternoon daylight supports more consistent and high-quality sleep. Raise the blinds to let in daylight or try to take a quick break outside. Even on cloudy days, natural light has a much stronger effect than indoor lighting.

2. Indulge in activities that make you use your muscles

Get up and move more often throughout the day. Choose to exercise in the late afternoon or early evening.

3. Take care of what you eat and drink in the evening and at night

Try eliminating high-sodium foods for dinner. Keep low on late-night snacking too. Assure adequate daytime fluid intake, and limit nighttime fluids. Eliminate nighttime caffeinated beverages. Avoid alcohol within three hours of bedtime.[187]

4. Don't drink alcohol at the end of the night.

Although alcohol can make you feel sleepy, it disrupts your sleep cycle and can make sleep less restorative. In addition, alcohol intake can lead to low blood sugar at night for diabetics (this is because the liver prioritizes breaking down alcohol instead of producing glucose via gluconeogenesis).

5. Establish a sleep schedule.

Start by ensuring you're allocating enough time each night to get at least seven hours of sleep, and then attempt to keep the same bedtime and wake-up time every day. It's alright if you can't follow this schedule perfectly or want to sleep a bit extra on the weekend, but you should aim to keep variations within a one-hour difference from your planned schedule.

6. Create a Sleep-Friendly Bedroom

A cool, dark, and quiet bedroom is most conducive to sleep. Set your thermostat to a comfortable temperature, and if you can't eliminate the sources of light and noise, consider blocking them out with earplugs and a sleep mask.

7. Avoid screen time for as long as you can before bed.

Electronics provoke mental stimulation that makes it more difficult to fall asleep. They also emit blue light that can throw off the body's system for inducing sleep. An hour without screen time before bed is ideal, but you can first try it for 10 or 20 minutes and build up from there.

Stress, Anxiety and Blood Glucose

When you first found out you had diabetes, you may have tested your blood glucose often and quickly figured out the influence of medications, diet, and activity on your glucose variability. But then—bam! Something made your blood sugar zoom up. And it didn't have anything to do with food, activity, or insulin.

What is it that can tear down all your carefully crafted glucose control? In a word—stress!

Stress is how your body and mind react to new or difficult situations. It might be short-term, like worrying about a presentation you're giving at work the next day. Or going to a party where you don't know many people at the weekend. It can also be something physical, like an accident or illness.

Living with diabetes itself can be stressful, and there can often be acute short-term stresses like an argument with your spouse, criticism from the boss or an unexpected traffic jam. However, these acute episodes can turn into chronic stress if they persist for a long time. For instance, if you are having to face bad traffic every day as you go to the office, or you're in a bad relationship with your spouse or a toxic work environment.

Chronic stress is a consistent sense of feeling pressured and overwhelmed over a long period. Both types of stress have a profound influence on your blood glucose.

If you're feeling stressed, your body releases stress hormones like cortisol and adrenaline. We produce these hormones as part of our body's defense system, known as the 'fight or flight' response, which increases insulin resistance. As it becomes tough for glucose to enter your cells, your blood glucose levels rise. It makes sense, right?

The thing your body needs to either fight or run away is energy. And therefore, it will use the energy available in your blood—the increased glucose.

But what if you don't need glucose? In most cases of acute stress in the modern world, you don't actually need to fight or run away and therefore you are not using up that glucose. More worrying than that is long—term stress. If stress doesn't go away, your blood sugar levels are likely to remain high, putting you at greater risk for diabetes, or if you already have diabetes, causing complications that affect the heart, nerves, and kidneys.

We do not have enough research to say that stress causes diabetes, as the link between stress and diabetes is complex and multifactorial. An interesting fact though, is that stress and depression are found to co-exist with diabetes, which means that people with diabetes are also reported to be more stressed and depressed compared to healthy individuals.

Stress and Diabetes

Everyone has stress in their lives. However, stress management for people with diabetes isn't just about finding ways to relax; it's also about managing blood glucose levels.

Diabetes is often a cause of stress, particularly in the early days when you've just been diagnosed. Paying close attention to what you eat and having many new things to learn and remember can feel overwhelming. Worrying about what the results will say or feeling anxious about needles can be really stressful.

You might hear about this thing called hypo anxiety where you stress about having a hypo episode. You might also feel guilty if the way they manage your diabetes goes off track, which is another stress factor!

If you feel this way from time to time, it's known as diabetes distress, and you're not alone. Research has shown that about 20-45% of adults with diabetes experience diabetes stress. If you don't manage this distress, things can worsen and lead to burnout.[188]

Ignoring stress or pretending it does not exist does not help. Using alcohol, cigarettes or other substances to cope with stress can harm your health and make it harder to manage diabetes.

Instead, indulging in self-management techniques related to your lifestyle can help to cope with this pressure.

Self-Management techniques that help you in coping with stress:

1. Cognitive Behavioural Therapy

Cognitive behavioural therapy, commonly known as CBT, was developed by the psychiatrist Aaron Beck in the 1960s. It is an evidence-based (supported by research) psychotherapeutic treatment with promising results in people with diabetes.

But what is it all about? Imagine this scenario. You're driving to your office in the morning—excited to start your day. Suddenly, your brain is consumed with an unwanted, disturbing thought about work, colleagues, or your boss. You continue to dwell on that thought throughout your drive. Have you ever experienced a similar scenario where an unwelcome thought seemingly appeared out of nowhere?

Do these thoughts make you sad, angry, agitated, or anxious and eventually influence your mood and behaviour? This is nothing unusual, but if this is happening often and you are getting trapped in this imaginary vicious cycle, you need to be reading about CBT therapy.

Cognitive behavioural therapy helps people learn how to identify and change destructive or disturbing thought patterns that negatively influence their behaviour and emotions. Through CBT, faulty thoughts are identified, challenged, and replaced with more objective, realistic thoughts.

Here is a 3-step technique for using CBT to manage your diabetes:

Step 1: What thoughts do you notice running through your mind concerning diabetes?

Be mindful of your thoughts related to diabetes; you could use your journal to list your common thoughts. They could be:

"This could destroy my life."

"I cannot live a happy life again."

"I cannot prevent complications."

Step 2: Challenge your thoughts by asking yourself:

"What is the evidence for and against this thought?"

"Is thinking this way helping me?"

For instance, if you think, "I cannot prevent complications," educate yourself with reliable scientific resources which show that you can indeed prevent complications.

Step 3: Think of an Alternative, Balanced Thought

Once you figure out the truth in your thought, you can decide on an action, however small or big, and move out of the negative thought pattern.

Here are some ways you can manage stress:

1. **Social Connectivity**: Close relationships with family and friends, frequent social interactions, talking out to someone you trust, getting help instead of trying to do everything yourself, joining a support group or online community for a cause, all these contribute to the downregulation of your

"fight and flight" response and nurture relaxing responses. Contributing to better glucose control and a longer healthier life.

A study from the Netherlands on 2000 plus participants found that isolated women lacking social participation had 112% higher odds of previously diagnosed type 2 diabetes than women with larger social networks. And withdrawn men with fewer social connections were 42% more likely to have previously been diagnosed with type 2 diabetes.[189]

Never discount the power of consistent small positive interactions. Smile at strangers. Ask work colleagues how they are, or what they did at the weekend.

2. **Positive Psychology**: Positive Psychology is the scientific study of the factors that enable individuals and communities to flourish, developed by an American Psychologist named Martin Seligman. It emphasises the positive effect of contentment with the past, happiness in the present and hope for the future. Its five building blocks, aka PERMA, are:
    i. Positive Emotion
    ii. Engagement
    iii. Relationships
    iv. Meaning
    v. Accomplishment

PERMA focuses on producing happiness, not lessening misery. Research studies have revealed that people with diabetes scored lower on overall PERMA dimensions of positive well-being than non-diabetics, implying the need to include activities that boost

PERMA to build resilience and effective coping skills.[190] For instance:

- Being mindful of everyday experiences like eating, tasting, smelling, and observing, and finding pleasure in those activities.
- Writing a daily gratitude journal and actively expressing your gratitude in words and actions.
- Kindness is a trait all happy people possess. Studies have shown that happiness and kindness go hand in hand and complement each other. Buy someone a small token of love or friendship, volunteer for a noble cause, donate something you don't need or use anymore or help a stranger in need. Kindness reinforces happiness and positivity.
- Healthy social bonds—personal and professional—are essential for happiness and inner peace. Being empathetic is foundational in forming healthy social bonds.[191]
- Optimistic interventions create positive outcomes by setting realistic expectations. An example of an optimistic PPI is the 'Imagine Yourself' test, where participants are asked to note down where they see themselves in the future.
- "It is within yourself that you will find the strength you need." Having a sense of self-worth and self-awareness can reduce the symptoms of depression and improve your self-esteem.
- Meaning-oriented positive psychology emphasises understanding and finding life's true meaning. So, activities like setting realistic goals and employing effective actions to achieve them, or just reflecting on our thoughts and emotions, could more likely make you feel happier and contented.[192]

Simple Self-Help Skills to Manage Stress

- Talk to someone you trust about your stress!
- Practice mindfulness, relaxation therapy, meditation, and breathing exercises.
- Find ways to laugh and spend time with people you enjoy.
- Get help instead of trying to do everything yourself.
- Spiritual and religious activities.
- Spend time in nature.
- Indulge in self-help books, websites, workshops and apps.
- Involve in volunteering for a meaningful cause.
- Do not put yourself down, have self-compassion.

Are stress and food related?

When you're under stress, finding ways to deal with it is natural. Some people binge-watch television, some smoke, and others turn to food. Finding solace in something—anything—is a way to block out or numb yourself to stress. Not many people reach for carrots or cucumbers when stressed; instead, they tend to turn to high carbohydrate and/or high-fat foods, such as ice cream, cookies, cake, or potato chips. Why carbs? These foods raise the levels of "feel good" brain chemicals, such as serotonin, dopamine, and endorphins.

There's a definite connection between stress and our appetite, but that connection isn't the same for everyone; some people overeat when they feel stressed, and others lose their appetite. Those who stop eating are so focused on their stress that they don't notice their hunger cues. Those who overeat are attempting to distract themselves with food. When stressed, your body releases the stress hormone cortisol. Cortisol can make you crave sugary, salty, and fatty foods because your brain thinks it needs fuel to fight whatever threat is causing the stress.[193]

The daily demands of work and home life and even the constant presence of electronic devices put people at high risk for stress eating. There is enough evidence to say that stress induces our eating choices, the amount of food we eat and how often.

The best way to combat stress or emotional eating is to be mindful of what triggers stress eating and to be ready to fight the urge. Refer to Chapter 5 for tips on mindful eating.

How does exercise reduce stress, and can exercise really be relaxing?

Exercise can relieve stress in almost any form. Being active boosts feel-good endorphins and distracts you from everyday worries. Physical movement is a substitute for insulin in the body and has some direct stress-busting benefits.

In short - it makes you feel better.

Exercise pumps up your endorphin levels, which helps you:

- Feel more confident
- Improve your mood
- Relax
- Cope with mild depression and anxiety
- Sleep better

It is meditation in motion.

Have you ever noticed when exercising, whether that is a walk in nature or at the gym, swimming or cycling, how you can lose track of time? You start getting more positive, productive thoughts which boost your self-esteem. In short, you have achieved the same results as meditation and added the physical health benefit.

It gives the opportunity to interact, socialise and make friends.

Social interactions have a profound effect on mental well-being. Exercise and sports allow you to get away from your daily schedule; as a result, you can find some time to enjoy solitude or interact with new people, make connections, and build a network.

Exercise is play and recreation. When your body is busy, your mind will be distracted from the worries of daily life and will be free to think creatively.

Even something as simple as taking deep breaths is a quick and easy way to calm down. Progressive relaxation focuses on tightening and relaxing specific muscle groups to both physically and mentally relax you.

Take Home Messages

- Getting active, prioritizing sufficient sleep, and practicing relaxation techniques can reduce bad cholesterol, strengthen your bones and muscles, improve your immunity, relieve stress, help you think clearly, improve your personal relationships, and keep your blood glucose in check.
- Active movement is about finding something that you love to do and that causes you to break a sweat.
- Through regular physical activity, blood glucose levels can be lowered by increasing muscle mass, reducing body fat,

improving mitochondrial function, and decreasing insulin requirements.
- The magic number for metabolically optimised sleep appears to be between seven to eight hours per night.
- Chronic stress can negatively impact blood glucose control and increase the risk of developing diabetes or worsening its symptoms. Managing stress through relaxation techniques and self-care can play a vital role in diabetes management.

CHAPTER 9

THE 5TH C- CAPITALISE ON TECHNOLOGY

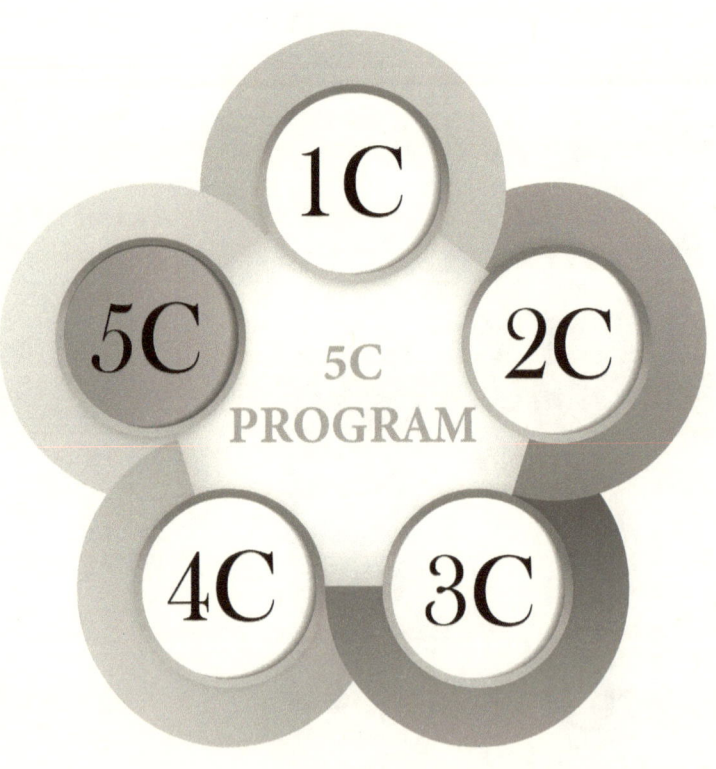

The 5th C- Capitalise on Technology

𝒴ou are now on a journey towards living a happy, healthy life. You now know how to move forward; you just need to keep your headlights on. What do I mean by that? Here's the thing, just like how headlights let you see where you're going in the dark, self-monitoring on a regular basis lets you see how certain foods, medications, and behaviours impact your health.

Today's world is full of devices, gadgets and healthcare solutions that help you to monitor yourself with ease and convenience. Diabetes is a persistent disease that needs to be continuously monitored. Your food, exercise and medication all need factoring in. A variety of medical devices have been developed to support lifestyle and pharmacological interventions (blood glucose meters, continuous glucose monitoring devices [CGM], insulin pumps, and smart pens) powered by technological advances.[194]

Technology is changing the way we live our lives and here you can find out how to manage your diabetes with technology. It may be best to track only one tool at a time and build slowly but surely so as not to be overwhelmed by these tools.

Most importantly, diabetes self-care technology must be personalised, you need to figure out what system is *your* system. And this largely depends on the type of diabetes you are tracking.

Table 9.1 Indicators to monitor based on medical condition

Condition	Indicators to Monitor
Prediabetes	Fasting blood glucose, Body weight, calories, activity
Type 2 Diabetes	Fasting and pre-2-hour post-meal glucose, carbohydrates, activity, sleep, blood pressure, heart rate
Type 1 Diabetes	Carbohydrates, insulin, activity, sleep, pre-2-hour post-meal glucose, hypoglycaemia
Gestational Diabetes	Weight gain, calorie intake, activity, pre-1-hour post-meal glucose
Polycystic ovarian syndrome	Body weight, calories, activity, menstrual cycle

Technology for checking blood glucose.
Glucometers

Home glucose monitors can help you keep tabs on your diabetes and lower your risk of complications. Along with treatment, using a home monitor can help you identify the things that make your blood sugar increase or decrease, from exercise to illness, stress to dehydration, and more.

The most important device for someone with diabetes to have is a glucometer. After a quick finger prick, you'll know your blood sugar level at that particular point in time. Even if you use a continuous glucose monitor (CGM), you'll still need a meter from time to time to confirm that the CGM readings are accurate

While nothing will be as accurate as a lab test, home tests can help provide peace of mind as well as better diabetes management. Here are a few things to consider when selecting a glucometer:

- Can you easily share data with your healthcare providers?
- Can you track other things like insulin, carb intake, and exercise?
- Can you make notes for each reading?
- How user-friendly is it?

Continuous Glucose Monitoring (CGM) Device

Continuous glucose monitoring has become an increasingly available choice for self-monitoring glucose levels over an extended period—and it can be highly effective. In Chapter 7, we discussed this device, but to summarise briefly,

- A small sensor is placed just under your skin, usually on your belly or arm. It is easy and quick to do this. In order to keep the sensor in place, adhesive tape is used.
- The sensor measures glucose levels in the fluid under your skin. Most CGM devices take readings every five minutes, all day and night. You'll need to change the sensor regularly based on the device. For most devices, you change sensors at home every 7 to 14 days.
- In all CGM systems, glucose information is wirelessly sent from the sensor to a device for viewing.

- Depending on the type of CGM, the data from the sensor is either transmitted to a handheld device called a receiver (similar to a cell phone), a smartphone app or an insulin pump.
- The real-time CGM system sends data continuously to the receiver and you can download CGM data (real-time glucose levels, trends, and history) to a computer anytime, whereas with a flash CGM, it's only when you wave (scan) your device over your sensor that you get your blood sugar readings.

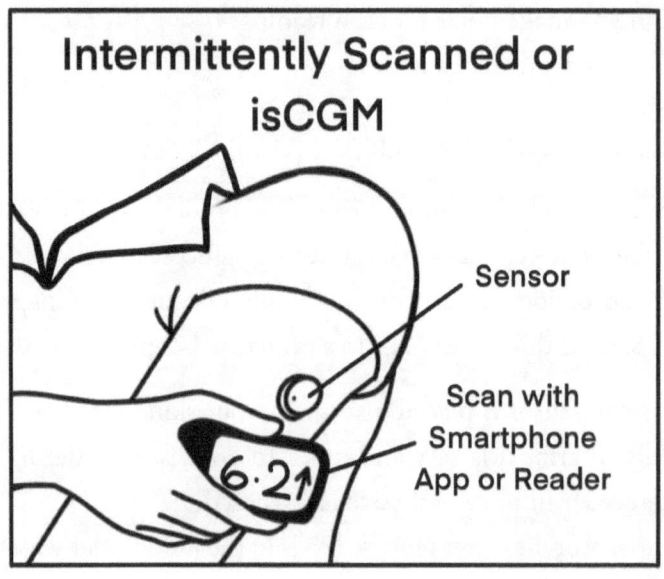

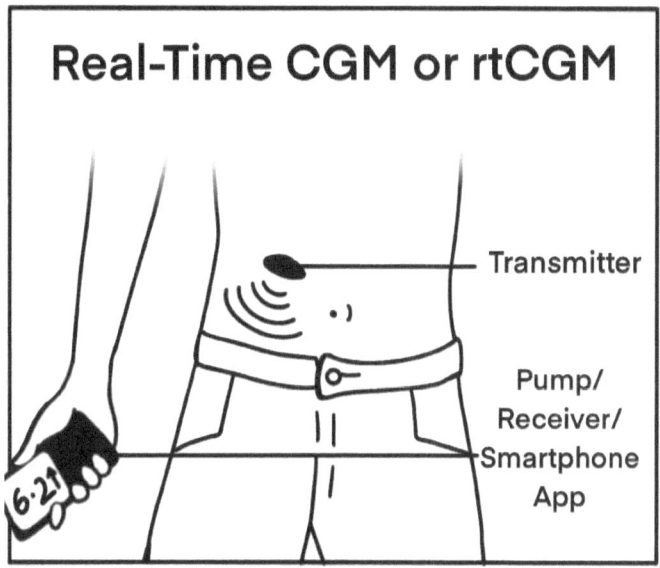

Among the remarkable advances in diabetes technology witnessed by the diabetes community in the past decade, CGM is having the greatest impact. CGM devices have become smaller, more affordable, more accurate, and more user-friendly.

A growing number of people with diabetes are using CGMs, especially those with type 1 diabetes, and where more meaningful targets for diabetes management such as time in range (TIR), time in hypoglycaemia, and blood glucose variability can be monitored than HbA1c alone. HbA1c indicates average blood glucose levels, but the fluctuations go undetected, which has a detrimental effect on the quality of life in people with type 1 diabetes.[195]

It takes time and patience to understand how a CGM device works. But you don't have to do it alone, a qualified professional can help you learn how to use it safely.

Technology to Manage your Diabetes.
Apps

One of your best health tools could be something you may already have - your cell phone.

If you have diabetes, you can download a diabetes management app. The key is finding the right app that addresses your concerns and makes managing your diabetes easier.

When choosing an app, look for features that address most of the diabetes management criteria you need, check table 9.1. Be sure to check these aspects as well.

- **An app that developers update regularly**. If it's not updated at some point, it won't work anymore.
- **User-friendly features**. If it is hard to understand you won't use it!
- **Integration with your other devices**. Some apps will integrate with your insulin pump, smartwatch, or other high-tech tools you may use to manage your diabetes. These can be time-saving and enhance how you manage your health.

Some apps allow you to share your health data with your medical team so that your doctors can help you make changes to your treatment regimen. Nowadays, diabetes apps can track blood sugar levels, provide trends, help you log your exercise, and connect you with other people who have diabetes for social support. A coaching app can also provide you with access to highly trained diabetes educators, nutritionists, and fitness coaches.

But it's important to check with your trusted diabetes health professional before you choose any app. An article published in

January 2020 in the journal 'Diabetes Care' noted that there isn't sufficient evidence to back up the effectiveness, accuracy, and safety of many apps, and many are plagued by technical problems.

The authors noted that regulatory agencies and app companies urgently need to work with diabetes health professionals and researchers to ensure the safety and effectiveness of diabetes apps.[196]

There are quite a few diabetes apps available for free. Whether you have an Android or an iPhone, the chances are that there is an app that will meet your needs. Be aware—free apps tend to have ads on them. And check the terms of the app as some may sell on your data.

Here is a list of a few that have been reviewed as best diabetes apps in 2022-23:

Fooducate, MySugr, Glucose Buddy, Beat Diabetes, Glucose Buddy, OneTouch Reveal, Glucose tracker—Diabetic diary, Diabetes, myfitnesspal, and calorieking.

It might also be worthwhile to explore regional applications that track calories and carbohydrates, as foods vary considerably by region and culture.

Fitness trackers

By tracking steps and the calories, you burn, fitness trackers can help anyone get fitter. But they have special benefits for people with diabetes. You will be motivated and pushed to achieve your targets using these trackers, which will improve your glucose control. It is worth repeating that even a small weight loss of 5 percent can result in a significant reduction in insulin resistance.

With most fitness trackers you can enter what you've eaten, or plan to eat, and it will show you the calories. They also balance the calories you burn with the ones you eat, so if you work out, you can indulge a bit more. Depending on your device and app, you can track your carbohydrates and insulin doses, so you can see all your data at once in easy-to-read graphs.

Smart Watches:

What exactly can a smartwatch do? Many have integrated all the functionality of fitness trackers. Health-related benefits include tracking your steps, heart rate, sleep quality, activity and overall fitness level.

Smart watches also measure the hours slept and quality of sleep, different manufacturers use different algorithms for tracking sleep time and quality with different levels of success. The better ones are able to know precisely when you have fallen asleep and woken up. Some of them also give you recommendations and reminders.

They often come with heart rate monitors that can measure your heart rate from the wrist. Measuring your heart rate has many benefits. You can track your heart rate during exercise allowing you to keep in a zone that's increasing your fitness level.

Another benefit is that heart rate measurement connected to Artificial Intelligence might be able to accurately detect specific types of abnormal heart rhythms. Your resting heart rate measurement is also an indication of your general fitness level, and some devices even do your fitness age based on your measurements.

Electrocardiogram (ECG) is a feature which is starting to be available on some smartwatches like the Apple Watch Series 4. It gives you more accurate heart rate measurements and gives more data for detecting possible heart-related problems.

Blood Pressure measurement is an entirely new feature for smartwatches. Passive blood pressure monitoring would allow individuals to see how their lifestyle affects their readings. It could help people make more informed choices about their diet and daily activities and ultimately help them reduce the risk of serious illness.

However, although there is great interest in monitoring blood pressure using wearables, this method has not yet been properly validated. Wrist measurements have so far failed to prove as accurate as those from a cuff.

There are apps that come pre-installed on some Smart Watches that send you reminders to stop and breathe. Some of these apps include options like setting the number of times your watch sends you reminders each day to stop and breathe and guided breathing practices that can range from 1 to 5 minutes to help you calm down, relax, and step into the present moment. When you stop and breathe, you can also help to lower your heart rate.

Smart watches can also be set to alert someone if you fall or have an accident, which can be reassuring if you have mobility issues.

Smart Insulin pens

Insulin pens are widely used to deliver subcutaneous insulin from a cartridge via a disposable needle. In spite of the convenience of this approach to insulin administration, the need to keep manual blood glucose readings make things challenging for healthcare professionals and users.

Over the last decade, insulin pen design has evolved to incorporate memory functions, caps, attachments, and now "smart insulin pens" that can track doses and upload data online. The "memory" function of the insulin pen, which stores and displays timings and amounts, is particularly useful for people who have difficulty sticking to a complex insulin regimen.

Using Bluetooth-enabled insulin pen caps and attachments, users can track everything.

Healthcare professionals can remotely review and adjust therapy with smart insulin pens because they can combine the above features with CGM data and upload it to online platforms. Smart pens may be an effective way to identify those who need education and support with behaviour modification at an earlier stage.

Studies in the T1D population have shown increased dosing adherence and better glucose control with smart pen use.[197] (Wang)

Who is a good candidate for using a smart pen?

Anyone with diabetes who:

- Uses multiple daily injections (MDI) and has access to a compatible smart phone and app.
- Struggles to calculate doses accurately, especially before meal doses based on meal carbohydrates. A bolus calculator feature available with smart pen technology makes it easy after you plug in the numbers.
- Misses doses and/or forgets when the last dose was. Data logging is done automatically and transmitted to the reading app on your smart phone.
- A person with type 1 diabetes who does not wish to use an insulin pump, but wants access to more detailed information regarding their insulin dose and glucose levels

Insulin pumps

Insulin pump therapy is one of the most notable advancements in diabetes technology in the past 50 years. Insulin pumps are battery-powered, electronic devices about the size of a cell phone that deliver insulin through a thin tube under the skin based on your body's needs throughout the day and night. Inside the pump is a vial of insulin with a gear-driven plunger, this is connected to a thin plastic tube, and the other end of the tube is a needle. You insert the needle under your skin, usually in areas of fat deposits like the abdomen or thigh. It's an alternative to frequent insulin injections, and some pumps can communicate with CGMs that track your blood glucose levels, too.

An insulin pump is intended to imitate the functions of a human pancreas. Your pancreas releases insulin in response to changes in your blood glucose level. But when you have diabetes, your body doesn't release insulin or use it properly. As a result, you have to find another way to get the insulin you need. You program the pump and give it instructions on how much insulin you want throughout the day and night (basal). Then, before each meal, you tell the pump how much insulin you need based on the carbohydrates in the meal (bolus).

You wear an insulin pump pretty much all the time, even when sleeping, showering or playing and even if you are swimming.

If needed, you can remove the pump, but be careful to put it back in within 1 hour. The other option is to go back to multiple daily injections with pens/syringes. Remember to keep your healthcare professional informed of any changes.

The right pump for you depends on what type of diabetes you have, your insurance status, and your age. Some pumps are not approved for children. It's important to talk with your doctor about choosing a pump. This can ensure the pump is the right option for you, your insulin needs, and your lifestyle.

Examples of commonly used insulin pumps today from Medtronic, Roche, Omnipod and Tandem.

What can the pump do for you?

- Ensure your blood sugar levels are close to normal by estimating how much insulin you will need during the day, at night, and before meals.
- Blood glucose fluctuations caused by inadequate and excessive insulin doses are reduced by this therapy.
- You can schedule the release of insulin based on your needs into specific time periods to deal with night-time lows and morning highs.

In insulin pump therapy, there is no one-size-fits-all approach. In recent years, insulin pump technology has advanced at an extraordinary rate, and it has the potential to improve diabetes outcomes for individuals of any age with type 1 or type 2 diabetes. Nevertheless, for insulin pump therapy to be successful, you must be able to overcome any barriers, have realistic expectations of the device, and perform self-care as well as complete comprehensive education and clinical follow-up.[198]

It is clear that smart technology can drastically improve and ease your life, by helping you to make informed decisions. Not only does it reduce the pain of pinching, pricking, and injecting insulin, but it gives you the power to make decisions about your management with your healthcare team.

Smart technology also promotes mindfulness in making daily life decisions, the discipline for self-management and self-care, and the formation of health habits. When you self-track, you see the rewards of your healthy habits. That can give you the motivation to stick with them. Not only can this help prevent or reduce the progression of diabetes and its complications, but it also can help reduce the costs of diabetes treatment and management.

I'm sure you're eager to put everything you've learned into practice. I'd like to give you a glimpse of how this might work for you as a 7-day plan to jumpstart applying what you've learned into practice.

In the meal plans, you will see that the food groups are highlighted. The purpose of these plans is to demonstrate how to mix food groups, make a healthy plate pattern, and maintain the right portion sizes and proportions.

Conclusion

I hope that I have been able to persuade you that diet, activity, sleep, and stress management are not stale clichés but actually the keys to not only diabetes control but to health in general. Several research scientists have invested years into unravelling the truth about diseases like diabetes, and in turn revealing the secret that the cure lies in its cause, namely a healthy lifestyle choice.

The goal of my book is to empower you and inspire you to make informed decisions, but at the end of the day, the choice is yours. However, you should know that there is only one way out of this sticky situation and that is the right lifestyle.

And there is only one person who can do that for you—and that is YOU.

Remember that there's no race to lose or competition to fail. The more you practice new skills and habits, the easier and more comfortable they become until this just becomes the way you live.

A healthy diet is not about eliminating certain foods from your diet. It's about eating whole real food in the right portions and proportions. It is not about what you do once but about what you do the majority of the time.

Lifestyle changes often fail because someone does something 'wrong' once and then thinks, 'I have ruined it now so I might as well not bother'. Don't be 'all or nothing.' Every small step you take towards better health is a good thing.

I don't know a single person who never eats something they 'shouldn't', or always gets their exercise in for the day—myself included. But it is what you do next that matters. Decide to keep going, to get back on track, and your future self will thank you for it.

Moreover, work towards fulfilling your life on all levels. Make sure you take the time to care for yourself and do whatever it takes to make yourself happy. Take time to just have fun. Take control of your life and live it to the fullest! Success will then follow.

Do visit my website for updated blogs and videos on these topics drsadiyalifestyle.com

APPENDIX I

Meal Plans

G-Grain	D-Dairy
V-Vegetables	P-Protein
F-Fruits	O-Oil/Fat

Day 1

Breakfast

1 slice Whole grain bread (G)
+ 1 tbsp. Nut butter (O)
+ 1 plum/ ½ c pomegranate (F)
+ 1 c Tea or coffee (no milk or sugar)

Lunch

2 c Chicken green pasta (G, P, V)
(Combine 1 c whole grain pasta with 2 c mixed vegetables, 60 gm chicken)

Snack

3 pcs Dark chocolate (O)
+ 1 c Herbal tea

Dinner

2 c Mixed bean salad (P, V, O)
(Combine 1c beans, 1 cup greens, ¼ c red onions, ½ c tomato slices, 2 tsp ground flaxseeds)
+ 2tbsp dressing (lime/vinegar/spices/mustard/olive oil)
+ 1 cup low-fat yoghurt with ¼ c berries (D, F)

Day 2

Breakfast

1 ½ c mixed fruits (F)
(Combine ½ c Berries, ½ c Papaya, ½ c Kiwi)
+ 1 Graham cracker (G)
+ 30 g low-fat cheddar cheese (D)
+ 1 c tea or coffee (no milk or sugar)

Lunch

1 cup spinach soup (V)
+ Grilled turkey pita sandwich (G, P, V)
(Stuff 1 whole grain pita with 60g shredded grilled chicken, ½ avocado, chopped lettuce, tomato, onion, and cucumber)

Snack

Handful of roasted nuts (O)
+ 1 c Herbal tea or black coffee

Dinner

2c Sweet potato bake (G, V, O)
(Combine 1c sweet potato, 1 c quinoa, 1 c vegetable broth ¼ cup chopped onions, herbs, and 2 tsp olive oil)
+ 1 c Green salad (V)

Day 3

Breakfast

1 whole wheat chapati (G)

+ 1 c vegetable curry (V, O)

+ 1 c green sprouts (P)

+ 1 c Tea with milk (D)

Lunch

1 cup cooked rice (G)
+ 1 cup salad (V)
+ 1 c Vegetable curry (V, O)
+ ½ c grilled paneer (P)

Snack

Handful nuts and date (O, F)
+ Tea with milk

Dinner

2 c Sweet potato bake (G, V, O)
(Combine 1c sweet potato, 1 c quinoa, 1 c vegetables broth ¼ cup chopped onions, herbs, and 2 tsp olive oil)
+ 1 c Green salad (V)

Day 4

Breakfast

1 slice whole grain bread (G)
+ 1 Vegetable omelette (P, V)
+ 1 c Green tea/white tea

Lunch

1 c Cooked Rice (G)
+ 1 c Oriental salad with cottage cheese (V, P)
+ ½ c Dahl with seasoning (P)
+ 1 cup vegetable curry (V)

Snack

2 plums (F)
+ 1 c Herbal tea

Dinner

1 Whole grain Chapati (G)
+ ½ c chickpea curry (P, O)
+ 1 c Vegetable Raita (V)
(Combine ½ c low-fat yoghurt with chopped tomatoes, onion, Cucumber, cilantro, 1 tsp ground flaxseeds)

Day 5

Breakfast

1 bowl Oats porridge (G, D, F)
(Cook ½ c steel-cut oats, 1 c low-fat milk, 3 dates/apricots, 2 tsp chia seeds)
+ 1 c Cinnamon Tea

Lunch

1 cup cooked brown rice (G)
+ 60 g grilled Fish (P)
+ 2 c stir-fried Vegetable (V,O)

Snack

1 cup baby carrots with hummus dip (V, P)
+ 1 c herbal tea

Dinner

2c Lentil vegetable soup (P, V, O)
(Combine ¼ c lentil, ½ diced tomato, 1c diced zucchini, ¼ c Chopped Onion, herbs and 1 tsp olive oil)
+ 1 whole grain toast (G)

Day 6

Breakfast

1 c Fruit yoghurt (F, D, O)
(Combine 1 c sliced fruits, 1 c low-fat yoghurt, ¼ roasted crushed nuts)
+ 1 c Green Tea

Lunch

2 c bean salad with feta cheese and egg (P, D, V)
(Combine 1 c boiled mixed beans, 1 cup chopped vegetables, 30 g feta cheese, 1 boiled egg)

Snack

½ c Boiled sweet potato (V)
+2 tsp peanut butter (O)

Dinner

1 c cooked zesty rice Pilaf (G, V, O)
(Recipe in the appendix)
+ 1 c Green salad with vinaigrette (V)

Day 7

Breakfast

1 whole wheat wrap (G)
+ 1 c vegetable sambar (V)
+ ½ c coconut chutney (O)
+ 1 c Tea or coffee with low-fat milk (D)

Snack

1 c Spicy sprout salad (V)
(Recipe in appendix)

Lunch

1 c Parboiled rice (G)
+ 1 c Vegetable curry (V)
+ 60 g chicken garlic grill (P)
+ 1 c Cucumber cilantro salad (V)

Snack

2 c Popcorn (G)

+ 1 c Herbal tea

Dinner

2 c Spinach fruit salad (V, F)
(Top 2c baby spinach leaves with 1c chopped bell pepper ¼ cup walnuts and 1 cup mandarin orange sections, salt and lemon juice)
+ 1 bowl dal soup (P)

APPENDIX II

Recipes

Ironically, many people following healthy diets eat even more variety of meals and recipes than they did on their regular "unrestricted" diet. When searching for healthy recipes, you will find a million results. If you are overwhelmed, use region-based, cuisine-based, and ingredient-based healthy recipes. In your exploration of learning more recipes, you are sure to find regional and cultural recipes that are healthy and interesting.

As discussed in Chapter 6 be sure to have your go-to recipes ready with at least five main courses, four salads, three snacks, two sandwiches, and one dessert.

I have included a few recipes below that I believe are easy healthy and quick.

Vibrant Vegetable Frittata

Servers 4

1 c baby spinach

½ c diced tomatoes

½ c finely chopped red onions

¼ c chopped bell pepper (orange, red, yellow)

2 tbsp feta cheese

2 eggs

Herbs (cilantro or basil)

Ground salt, pepper, turmeric

1 tsp olive oil

1. Heat the oven to 180°C
2. Medium heat the sauté pan, and add olive oil/spray oil. Sauté spinach until wilted; remove from heat.
3. In a mixing bowl, whisk the egg until fluffy and gradually add all the ingredients; mix well.
4. Pour the mixture into the warm pan, stir it and cover with foil.
5. Bake for approximately 20 minutes in the oven or you may also use a microwave.
6. Cut into four squared and serve with whole grain toast and a cup of non-calorie tea or coffee.

Chicken salad sandwich

Serves 2

4 slices whole-grain bread or 2 small whole grain pitta bread

100 grams chicken breast (boneless and skinless)

1 tbsp white pepper

1 tbsp onion powder

¼ cup tahina sauce or hummus or Swiss cheese

½ cup lettuce

¼ cup sliced tomatoes

1. Heat oven to 180°C.
2. Season the chicken with salt, pepper and onion powder. Grill or bake until thoroughly cooked (you may also do a batch cooking and store in portions in the refrigerator for a quick sandwich).
3. In a medium bowl mix all diced chicken pieces with vegetables, spices and hummus/tahina/cheese. Refrigerate until ready to serve.
4. To build the sandwich, place about ½ cup chicken salad mixture on the slice of bread or fill it in the pita and grill it before your serve.

Zesty Rice Pilaf

Serves 2

1 c Rice, rinsed (preferably brown rice)

2 cups of finely chopped vegetables (onion, mushroom, tomato, carrot, broccoli)

2 cups home-made vegetable broth

Herbs and spices-garlic, cloves, pepper, turmeric

1. In a medium pan over medium heat, sauté onions until golden brown.
2. Add the vegetables and spices to cook until slightly soft.
3. Add the vegetable broth and wait until it boils.
4. Add the rice, cover and simmer over very low heat until the broth is absorbed and the rice is medium soft and done.
5. Serve with grilled chicken or cottage cheese.

Sweet potato bake

Serve 3

2 c sweet potatoes diced into small cubes

2 cups vegetable broth

½ cup chickpeas/black beans (cooked)

½ cup corn

1 tsp cumin powder

¼ tsp thyme

¼ cup chopped green onion

1. Preheat the oven to 180° C.
2. In a large baking dish, combine the sweet potatoes, broth, beans, quinoa, corn, cumin, chilli powder, and thyme.
3. Stir until mixed well and cover with foil.
4. Bake for 45 minutes.
5. Remove the foil and bake for an additional 15 to 20 min, or until most of the liquid has been absorbed and the potatoes are tender.
6. Let the dish sit for 5 min so any remaining liquid can be absorbed.
7. Sprinkle with the green onions and serve.

Cauliflower rice topped with dal

Serve 2

2 medium heads of cauliflower

1 medium white onion, diced

2 garlic cloves

2 cups homemade vegetable broth or chicken stock

3 c of home-made tomato paste

1 tbsp curry powder

2 c cooked lentils

1. Break up the cauliflower into individual florets and grind them in a manual food processor until they reach rice-like consistency and keep aside. Be careful not to overprocess or it will become mushy.
2. Heat saucepan on medium flame, add 2 tsp vegetable oil, add the onion and cook until golden brown, about 10-12 minutes.
3. Add crushed garlic and cook for 2 minutes, followed by tomato sauce and curry powder.
4. Pour the stock and mix well and reduce the heat to cook for 5-7 min.
5. Boiled dahl with salt, turmeric, and spices into a sauce.
6. Serve the cauliflower rice topped with dal and side it with a bowl of crunchy salad.

Spicy sprout salad

Serve 1

1 c sprout beans

¼ c spring onion chopped

2 tsp sesame oil/olive oil

2 garlic cloves grated or use garlic powder

½ tap toasted sesame seeds

½ tsp toasted flaxseeds

Salt

1. Mix all the ingredients in a medium bowl and serve with sparkling water lemon mint.

Date with oats

Serve 2

½ c steel-cut oats/old-fashioned oats

1 c low-fat milk (instead you may also use water)

5 dates cut into pieces

¼ tsp cinnamon powder

1. Mix the oats with milk in a saucepan, and bring to a boil.
2. Once the oats start to thicken, you may add the dates and cinnamon powder and stir for a minute.
3. Dig into a healthy breakfast.
4. Tip: you may make your own variations with fruits, milk, and spice flavours.

APPENDIX III

Monotherapy

Metformin (Biguanide)

Metformin falls under the drug class called Biguanides and is popular under the brand name Glucophage. Usually, when you are newly diagnosed with type 2 diabetes, your physician will start with monotherapy (treatment with one drug). Presently, all the guidelines recommend metformin as the first choice for initiating pharmacologic treatment in people with type 2 diabetes and titrating the dose from 500 to 2000 mg per day as tolerated with or after meals. Taking metformin reduces glucose production in the liver, increases the body's sensitivity to insulin, and decreases sugar absorption from the intestines. This drug also decreases appetite and, therefore, caloric intake, facilitating weight loss. However, it may block vitamin B12 absorption in the body over time. Your doctor will prescribe B12 vitamin supplements if necessary.[199]

Metformin is a go-to prescription drug for younger women dealing with diabetes and fertility issues. It controls the onset and worsening of polycystic ovary syndrome or PCOS.[200]

Dual Therapy

When monotherapy with metformin (or its replacement) is not sufficiently effective to reach the HbA1c target, or it fails afterward, a second glucose-lowering drug is recommended by all guidelines. Either of the medications is added based on guidelines. The list of medications includes:

DPP4 Inhibitors
- Sulfonylurea
- Glinides
- Pioglitazone
- Alpha-Glucosidase
- GLP1 Receptor Agonists
- SGLT2 Inhibitors

DPP-4 Inhibitors

These are all gliptins or Dipeptidyl peptidase-4 inhibitors(DPP-4), and you will find them in pharmacies such as Sitagliptin (Januvia), Vildagliptin (Galvus), Saxagliptin (Onglyza), Linagliptin (Tradjenta), and Gemigliptin (Zemiglo).

The hormone Glucagon is responsible for decreasing insulin (when insulin decreases, it increases glucose). It facilitates the movement of digested food from the stomach to the intestines for absorption, eventually increasing blood glucose. DPP-4 inhibitors work by blocking the action of DPP-4, an enzyme which destroys incretins such as GLP-1. Incretins provide slower gastric emptying and help the body produce more insulin only when it is needed and reduce the amount of glucose being produced by the liver when it is not needed.[201]

GLP-1 Agonists (Incretin Mimetics)

Glucagon-like peptide (GLP-1) agonist is an incretin mimic. Let us look at what 'Incretin Mimetics' means. Incretin is one of the hormones that play a major role in stimulating Insulin secretion and keeping your blood glucose level. They come from your gut, ideally after each meal. One of the most important effects of GLP1 is also to reduce hunger and increase satiety, which leads to weight loss. Stomach emptying also becomes slower, which can cause gastrointestinal side effects. The incretin hormone GLP-1 uniquely stimulates insulin and inhibits glucagon secretion, thereby lowering plasma glucose levels.[202]

The Three-Pronged Approach

GLP-1 agonists control blood sugar majorly through three functions:

i. GLP-1 agonists keep your food in the stomach for longer and prevent it from moving into the small intestines. This action slows down the digestion process, keeps you full for longer, and keeps blood glucose levels under check for a greater period of the day. The medication helps you take the reins of your appetite and weight loss journey by creating a better rapport between your brain and gut.[203]

ii. GLP-1 stimulates the release of insulin and consequently brings down blood glucose levels.

iii. When GLP-1 inhibitors are at work in your system, the liver cannot release sugars into your bloodstream beyond the restricting levels. It keeps a check on your fasting blood glucose as well.

The Options Available

GLP-1 inhibitors can be taken orally or by injections. They are available as short-acting (works for less than 24 hours, available as Exenatide (Byetta), Lixisenatide (Adlyxin), and Oral Semaglutide (Rybelsus), and long-acting GLP-1 inhibitors (works one day to one week), commonly prescribed as Dulaglutide (Trulicity), Exenatide Extended-Release (Bydureon), Liraglutide (Victoza), and Semaglutide (Ozempic).

This class of drugs also reduces your body fat content and is effectively used for weight loss in obese patients. Commonly prescribed with the name Saxenda (liraglutide) and Wegovy (semaglutide).

GIP receptor / GLP-1 receptor agonists

They work by lowering blood sugar levels by releasing insulin into the bloodstream and by reducing glucagon levels. Commonly prescribed with the name Mounjaro (Tirzepatid).

Alpha-Glucosidase Inhibitors

Alpha-glucosidase inhibitors or AGIs are oral medications routinely used in treating type 2 diabetes and impaired glucose tolerance. Commonly sold as acarbose (Precose) and miglitol (Glyset).

AGIs work vastly by slowing down the digestion and absorption of complex carbohydrates such as fibers and starches, plateauing the blood glucose levels after the meal.[204]

Our body does not absorb glucose only from the intestines. The starchy food we eat is fermented in the colon and used for energy (or metabolized). On top of controlling glucose levels at the beginning of digestion, alpha-glucosidase inhibitors lower these sugars' metabolic effects and reduce their bioavailability.

SGLT 2 Inhibitors

SGLT 2 Inhibitors, also known as gliflozins, improve blood sugar control in patients with type 2 diabetes. Available in pharmacies as Canagliflozin (Invokana), Dapagliflozin (Farxiga), Empagliflozin (Jardiance), Ertugliflozin (Steglatro), Ipragliflozin (Suglat), and Luseogliflozin (Lusefi). This drug class is also known to help weight loss and blood pressure regulation. In recent years, studies have shown that SGLT2 inhibitors reduce the risk of morbidity in heart failure and progression of kidney disease both in diabetics and in individuals without diabetes.

Our kidneys work by absorbing toxic molecules, waste products, unwanted salts, excess water, glucose, and other particles from our blood. When our body is short of water, certain salts (ions), or glucose, the kidneys may release small amounts into the body under the action of hormones (vasopressin, diuretic, et cetera). SGLT 2 inhibitors prevent the taking back of glucose, called renal glucose reabsorption.

Insulin Secretagogues

A secretagogue is any substance that causes a body part to secrete something. Insulin Secretagogues signal the beta-cells in the pancreas to secrete insulin. They are classified as Sulfonylureas and Nonsulfonylureas—both kinds may appear in your prescriptions.

Sulfonylureas

The first generation of the drug class includes glimepiride (amary) and glipizide (Glucitrol), and Glyburide (Diabeta). Sulfonylureas make your beta cells a little more insulin at any given blood glucose level (as long as beta cells in the pancreas are still able to make insulin). They may stop your liver from putting stored glucose into the blood. These actions reduce your blood glucose.

Non-sulfonylureas

We have already discussed the Non-sulfonylurea insulin secretagogues called biguanides and AGIs. Thiazolidinediones and Meglitinides (repaglinide and nateglinide) comprise other classes of nonsulfonylureas. The latter group is found to act rapidly and effectively against diabetes, while the effects are short-lived. Nonsulfonylureas notoriously increase body weight. This subgroup of drugs improves the action of insulin and delays the digestion of carbohydrates.

Thiazolidinediones - TZDs

Also known as Glitazones, you may come across Lobeglitazone (Duvie), Rosiglitazone (Avandia), Pioglitazone (Pioglit, Actos), and Troglitazone (Rezulin) in the prescriptions of a diabetic person. Thiazolidinediones or TZDs act essentially by increasing insulin sensitivity. They make a great candidate if you have multiple conditions, especially high blood pressure, although type 2 diabetes is the only approved indication.

Triple Therapy

A third glucose-lowering drug should be added if dual therapy is not sufficiently effective to reach or maintain the HbA1c target. The most common choice to add to two oral glucose-lowering drugs is basal insulin.GLP1 receptor agonist can be added instead if weight loss has been insufficient.

Injectables for Type 2 Diabetes

Injectable drugs are recommended for type 2 diabetes when oral medication therapies are insufficient or impracticable. GLP-1 agonists (discussed above), and insulin are the most common drugs that fight glucose toxicity related to type 2 diabetes.

(3) Insulins

Insulin is the crux of blood glucose control. With type 1, your pancreas doesn't make insulin anymore, or only a tiny amount. In either case, you need to take insulin. If you have type 2 diabetes, your pancreas may still make insulin, but not enough, so you may sometimes need to take insulin along with pills. Don't worry, taking insulin doesn't mean you're doing anything wrong with your diabetes care. Adhering to your doctor's recommendations is best.

Insulin's action has three parts: onset, peak and duration. Onset is how long insulin takes to start working. Peak is when insulin is working its hardest. Duration is how long it lasts before it stops working. The time of onset, peak and duration are given as ranges in the below table. The main reason for these ranges is that insulin may work slower or faster in you than in someone else.

Table 2.4: Insulin is delivered to the body in different forms.

	Types of Insulin and How They Work			
Insulin type	How fast does it start to work (onset)	Available as	When it peaks	How long it lasts (duration)
Rapid-acting	About 15 minutes after injection	Lispro (Humalog), Aspart (Novolog), Glulisine (Apidra)	1 hour	2 to 4 hours
Short-acting, also called regular	Within 30 minutes after injection	Regular ® or Novolin	2 to 3 hours	3 to 6 hours
Intermediate-acting	2 to 4 hours after injection	NPH ®	4 to 12 hours	12 to 18 hours

Types of Insulin and How They Work

Insulin type	How fast does it start to work (onset)	Available as	When it peaks	How long it lasts (duration)
Long-acting	Several hours after injection	Glargine (Lantus, Toujeo), Detemir (Levemir), Degludec (Tresiba)	Does not peak	24 hours; some last longer
Premixed*	30 minutes	Humulin 70/30	2-4 hours	Lasts up to 24 hours

*Premixed insulins combine specific amounts of intermediate-acting and short-acting insulin in one insulin pen.

i. If you are more familiar with NovoLog or the NovoLog FlexPen, you have 'Insulin Aspart,' a high-performer to be prescribed only by your doctor. It is taken before and after meals.
ii. Levemir acts for longer as it gives you 'Insulin detemir.' It is dosed once or twice a day.
iii. Lantus, Lantus Solostar, and Toujeo deliver 'Insulin glargine' and work just like 'Insulin detemir.'
iv. Humulin N and Novolin N consist of 'Insulin isophane,' intermediate-acting insulin. You mix it well before injecting it,

as it is a colloidal mixture. It is also called Neutral Protamine Hagedorn or NPH insulin.

v. Humulin 70/30 and Novolin 70/30 are 70% NPH insulin and 30% regular insulin (Insulin isophane 70% and insulin 30%). Since it is a mixture of intermediate-acting insulin with a short-acting one, it is prescribed only in special cases.

vi. If your doctor asks you to take Humalog, you have the rapid-acting insulin injection called 'Insulin Lispro.'

REFERENCES

Chapter 1

1. International Diabetes Federation: Facts and Figures. https://idf.org/aboutdiabetes/what-is-diabetes/facts-figures.html
2. Our World Data: Daily supply of calories per person, 2018. https://ourworldindata.org/grapher/daily-per-capita-caloric-supply
3. Hostalek, U. Global epidemiology of prediabetes - present and future perspectives. *Clin Diabetes Endocrinol* 5, 5 (2019). https://doi.org/10.1186/s40842-019-0080-0
4. Zong G, Eisenberg DM, Hu FB, Sun Q. Consumption of Meals Prepared at Home and Risk of Type 2 Diabetes: An Analysis of Two Prospective Cohort Studies. *PLoS Med*. 2016 Jul 5;13(7):e1002052. doi: 10.1371/journal.pmed.1002052. PMID: 27379673; PMCID: PMC4933392.
5. Koopman ADM, Beulens JW, Dijkstra T, et al. Prevalence of insomnia (symptoms) in T2D and association with metabolic parameters and glycemic control: meta-analysis. *J Clin Endocrinol Metab*. 2020;105(3):614–643. doi: 10.1210/clinem/dgz065
6. Schipper, S.B.J., Van Veen, M.M., Elders, P.J.M. et al. Sleep disorders in people with type 2 diabetes and associated health outcomes: a review of the literature. Diabetologia 64, 2367–2377 (2021). https://doi.org/10.1007/s00125-021-05541-0

Chapter 2

7. Guyton AC, Hall JE. Guyton and Hall Textbook of Medical Physiology. New York: Saunders/Elsevier; 2011.

8. Ralph A. DeFronzo, Roy Eldor, Muhammad Abdul-Ghani; Pathophysiologic Approach to Therapy in Patients With Newly Diagnosed Type 2 Diabetes. *Diabetes Care* 1 August 2013; 36 (Supplement_2): S127–S138. https://doi.org/10.2337/dcS13-2011
9. Chieh-Hua Lu, Teng Sen-Wen, Chung-Ze Wu, et al. The roles of first phase, second phase insulin secretion, insulin resistance, and glucose effectiveness of having prediabetes in nonobese old Chinese women. *Medicine* 99(12):p e19562, March 2020. | DOI: 10.1097/MD.0000000000019562
10. Parry SA, Rosqvist F, Mozes FE, et al. Intrahepatic fat and postprandial glycemia increase after consumption of a diet enriched in saturated fat compared with free sugars. *Diabetes Care* 2020; 43:1134–1141. doi: 10.2337/dc19-2331.
11. Sears, B., Perry, M. The role of fatty acids in insulin resistance. *Lipids Health Dis* 14, 121 (2015). https://doi.org/10.1186/s12944-015-0123-1
12. Capucho AM, Conde SV. Impact of Sugars on Hypothalamic Satiety Pathways and Its Contribution to Dysmetabolic States. *Diabetology*. 2023; 4(1):1-10. https://doi.org/10.3390/diabetology4010001
13. UKPDS. U.K. Prospective diabetes study 16. Overview of 6 years' therapy of type II diabetes: a progressive disease. U.K. Prospective diabetes study group. *Diabetes*. 1995 Nov;44(11):1249–1258.
14. International Diabetes Federation. IDF Diabetes Atlas, 8th ed. Brussels, Belgium: International Diabetes Federation; 2017.
15. Diabetes Prevention Program Research Group. Long-term effects of lifestyle intervention or metformin on diabetes development and microvascular complications over 15-year follow-up: the Diabetes Prevention Program Outcomes Study. *The Lancet Diabetes & Endocrinology*. 2015;3(11):866–875.
16. Hamman RF, Wing RR, Edelstein SL, et al. Effect of weight loss with lifestyle intervention on risk of diabetes. Diabetes Care. 2006 Sep;29(9):2102-7
17. Ramlo-Halsted BA, Edelman SV. The natural history of type 2 diabetes. Implications for clinical practice. Prim Care. 1999 Dec;26(4):771-89. doi: 10.1016/s0095-4543(05)70130-5.

18. Plows JF, Stanley JL, Baker PN, Reynolds CM, Vickers MH. The Pathophysiology of Gestational Diabetes Mellitus. Int J Mol Sci. 2018;19(11):3342.
19. Gestational Diabetes. International Diabetes Federation. Updated 7 Jan 2020. https://www.idf.org/our-activities/care-prevention/gdm. Accessed Feb 7, 2022.
20. Sadiya, A., Jakapure, V., Shaar, G, et al. Lifestyle intervention in early pregnancy can prevent gestational diabetes in high-risk pregnant women in the UAE: a randomized controlled trial. *BMC Pregnancy Childbirth* 22, 668 (2022). https://doi.org/10.1186/s12884-022-04972-w
21. Nkonge, K.M., Nkonge, D.K. & Nkonge, T.N. The epidemiology, molecular pathogenesis, diagnosis, and treatment of maturity-onset diabetes of the young (MODY). *Clin Diabetes Endocrinol* **6**, 20 (2020). https://doi.org/10.1186/s40842-020-00112-5
22. American Diabetes Association Professional Practice Committee; 2. Classification and Diagnosis of Diabetes: *Standards of Medical Care in Diabetes—2022. Diabetes Care* 1 January 2022; 45 (Supplement_1): S17–S38.
23. Riddle MC, Cefalu WT, Evans PH, et al. Consensus Report: Definition and Interpretation of Remission in Type 2 Diabetes. Diabetes Care. 2021 Aug 30;44(10):2438–44. doi: 10.2337/dci21-0034.
24. Bergman, M., Buysschaert, M., Medina, J.L. et al. Remission of T2DM requires early diagnosis and substantial weight reduction. *Nat Rev Endocrinol* 18, 329–330 (2022). https://doi.org/10.1038/s41574-022-00670-x
25. Esposito K, Maiorino MI, Bellastella G, Chiodini P, Panagiotakos D, Giugliano D. A journey into a Mediterranean diet and type 2 diabetes: a systematic review with meta-analyses. BMJ Open. 2015 Aug 10;5(8):e008222. doi: 10.1136/bmjopen-2015-008222
26. Wilding JPH, Batterham RL, Calanna S, et al. STEP 1 Study Group. Once-Weekly Semaglutide in Adults with Overweight or Obesity. *N Engl J Med.* 2021 Mar 18;384(11):989-1002. doi: 10.1056/NEJMoa2032183.

27. Jastreboff AM, Aronne LJ, Ahmad NN, et al. SURMOUNT-1 Investigators. Tirzepatide Once Weekly for the Treatment of Obesity. N Engl J Med. 2022 Jul 21;387(3):205-216. doi: 10.1056/NEJMoa2206038.
28. Moradi, M., Kabir, A., Khalili, D. et al. Type 2 diabetes remission after Roux-en-Y gastric bypass (RYGB), sleeve gastrectomy (SG), and one anastomosis gastric bypass (OAGB): results of the longitudinal assessment of bariatric surgery study. *BMC Endocr Disord* 22, 260 (2022). https://doi.org/10.1186/s12902-022-01171-8
29. Nuha A. ElSayed, Grazia Aleppo, et al. Pharmacologic Approaches to Glycemic Treatment: Standards of Care in Diabetes—2023. *Diabetes Care* 1 January 2023; 46 (Supplement_1): S140–S157. https://doi.org/10.2337/dc23-S009

Chapter 3

30. Ströhle A, Hahn A. Diets of modern hunter-gatherers vary substantially in their carbohydrate content depending on ecoenvironments: results from an ethnographic analysis. *Nutr Res*. 2011 Jun;31(6):429-35
31. Nantel G. Carbohydrates in human nutrition. FAO/WHO report. 1998 https://www.fao.org/3/x2650T/x2650t02.htm
32. Evert AB, Boucher JL, Cypress M, et al. Nutrition therapy recommendations for the management of adults with diabetes. *Diabetes Care* 2014;37(Suppl. 1):S120–S143
33. Alison B. Evert, Michelle Dennison, Christopher D. Gardner, et al. Nutrition Therapy for Adults With Diabetes or Prediabetes: A Consensus Report. *Diabetes Care* 1 May 2019; 42 (5): 731–754. https://doi.org/10.2337/dci19-0014
34. Schwingshackl L, Hoffmann G, Lampousi AM, et al. Food groups and risk of type 2 diabetes mellitus: a systematic review and meta-analysis of prospective studies. *Eur J Epidemiol*. 2017 May;32(5):363-375.
35. Huang Y, Chen Z, Chen B, Li J, Yuan X, Li J et al. Dietary sugar consumption and health: umbrella review *BMJ* 2023; 381 :e071609

36. Hu Y, Ding M, Sampson L, et al. Intake of whole grain foods and risk of type 2 diabetes: results from three prospective cohort studies. *BMJ.* 2020 Jul 8;370
37. Neuenschwander M, Ballon A, Weber KS, et al. Role of diet in type 2 diabetes incidence: umbrella review of meta-analyses of prospective observational studies. *BMJ.* 2019 Jul 3;366:l2368.
38. Reynolds A, Mann J, Cummings J, et al. Carbohydrate quality and human health: a series of systematic reviews and meta-analyses. Lancet. 2019 Feb 2;393(10170):434-445.
39. United States Department of Agriculture: Fooddata Central. https://fdc.nal.usda.gov/
40. Sanders LM, Allen JC, Blankenship J, etal. Implementing the 2020-2025 Dietary Guidelines for Americans: Recommendations for a path forward. *J Food Sci.* 2021 Dec;86(12):5087-5099
41. Canada#x2019s Food Guide. Ottawa: Health Canada; 2007.
42. Juntunen KS, Niskanen LK, Liukkonen KH, et al. Postprandial glucose, insulin, and incretin responses to grain products in healthy subjects. *Am J Clin Nutr.* 2002;75(2):254-262.
43. Gibney MJ, Vorster HH, Kok FJ, eds. *Introduction to human nutrition.* Oxford, UK: Blackwell Science, 2002:1–11.
44. Jenkins DJ, Wolever TM, Taylor RH, et al. Glycemic index of foods: a physiological basis for carbohydrate exchange. *Am J Clin Nutr.* 1981 Mar;34(3):362-6
45. Livesey G, Taylor R, Livesey H, Liu S. Is there a dose-response relation of dietary glycemic load to risk of type 2 diabetes? Meta-analysis of prospective cohort studies. Am J Clin Nutr. 2013;97:584-96.
46. Mirrahimi A, de Souza RJ, Chiavaroli L, et al. Associations of glycemic index and load with coronary heart disease events: a systematic review and meta-analysis of prospective cohorts. J Am Heart Assoc 2012;1
47. Risérus U, Willett WC, Hu FB. Dietary fats and prevention of type 2 diabetes. *Prog Lipid Res.* 2009 Jan;48(1):44-51.
48. Imamura F, Micha R, Wu JH, et al. Effects of Saturated Fat, Polyunsaturated Fat, Monounsaturated Fat, and Carbohydrate on

Glucose-Insulin Homeostasis: A Systematic Review and Meta-analysis of Randomised Controlled Feeding Trials. *PLoS Med.* 2016 Jul 19;13(7):

49. Mensink, R.P., et al., Effects of dietary fatty acids and carbohydrates on the ratio of serum total to HDL cholesterol and on serum lipids and apolipoproteins: a meta-analysis of 60 controlled trials. *Am J Clin Nutr*, 2003. 77(5): p. 1146-55.

50. Shai I, Schwarzfuchs D, Henkin Y, et al.; Dietary Intervention Randomized Controlled Trial (DIRECT) Group. Weight loss with a low-carbohydrate, Mediterranean, or low-fat diet. *N Engl J Med* 2008;359:229–241

51. Drouin-Chartier JP, Li Y, Ardisson Korat AV, et al. Changes in dairy product consumption and risk of type 2 diabetes: results from 3 large prospective cohorts of US men and women. *Am J Clin Nutr.* 2019 Nov 1;110(5):1201-1212

52. Mozaffarian, D., et al., Dietary intake of trans fatty acids and systemic inflammation in women. *Am J Clin Nutr*, 2004. 79(4): p. 606-12.

53. USDA National Nutrient Databse-Cholesterol: https://www.nal.usda.gov/sites/default/files/page-files/cholesterol.pdf

54. Peterman MG. The ketogenic diet in the treatment of epilepsy: a preliminary report. *American journal of diseases of children.* 1924 Jul 1;28(1):28-33.

55. Goday A, Bellido D, Sajoux I, et al. Short-term safety, tolerability and efficacy of a very low-calorie-ketogenic diet interventional weight loss program versus hypocaloric diet in patients with type 2 diabetes mellitus. *Nutrition & diabetes.* 2016 Sep;6(9):e230-.

56. Heli E K Virtanen, Sari Voutilainen, Timo T Koskinen, et al. Dietary proteins and protein sources and risk of death: the Kuopio Ischaemic Heart Disease Risk Factor Study. *Am J Clin Nutr* , 2019; DOI: 10.1093/ajcn/nqz025

57. Annalisa Giosuè, Ilaria Calabrese, Gabriele Riccardi, Olga Vaccaro, Marilena Vitale, Consumption of different animal-based foods and risk of type 2 diabetes: An umbrella review of meta-analyses of prospective studies, *Diabetes Research and Clinical Practice*, Volume 191,2022, https://doi.org/10.1016/j.diabres.2022.110071.

58. Christopher D Gardner et al. Effect of a ketogenic diet versus Mediterranean diet on glycated hemoglobin in individuals with prediabetes and type 2 diabetes mellitus: The interventional Keto-Med randomized crossover trial, *The American Journal of Clinical Nutrition*, Volume 116, Issue 3, September 2022, Pages 640–652

Chapter 4

59. Global Burden of Disease Collaborative Network. Global Burden of Disease Study 2019. Results. Institute for Health Metrics and Evaluation. 2020 (https://vizhub.healthdata.org/gbd-results/)
60. de Boer IH, Bangalore S, Benetos A, et al. Diabetes and hypertension: a position statement by the American Diabetes Association. *Diabetes Care* 2017;40:1273–1284
61. Zhu P, Pan XF, Sheng L, Chen H, Pan A. Cigarette Smoking, Diabetes, and Diabetes Complications: Call for Urgent Action. *Curr Diab Rep*. 2017 Sep;17(9):78. doi: 10.1007/s11892-017-0903-2.
62. Nuha A. ElSayed, Grazia Aleppo, et al. Glycemic Targets: Standards of Care in Diabetes—2023. *Diabetes Care* 1 January 2023; 46 (Supplement_1): S97–S110. https://doi.org/10.2337/dc23-S006
63. Purnell, J. Q., Zinman, B., Brunzell, J. D., & DCCT/EDIC Research Group (2013). The effect of excess weight gain with intensive diabetes mellitus treatment on cardiovascular disease risk factors and atherosclerosis in type 1 diabetes mellitus results from the Diabetes Control and Complications Trial/Epidemiology of Diabetes Interventions and Complications Study (DCCT/EDIC) study. *Circulation*, 127(2), 180–187. https //doi.org/10.1161/CIRCULATIONAHA.111.077487
64. Nathan DM; DCCT/EDIC Research Group. The diabetes control and complications trial/epidemiology of diabetes interventions and complications study at 30 years overview. *Diabetes Care*. 2014;37(1) 9-16. doi 10.2337/dc13-2112.
65. UK Prospective Diabetes Study (UKPDS) Group (1998) Intensive blood-glucose control with sulphonylureas or insulin compared with conventional treatment and risk of complications in patients with type

2 diabetes (UKPDS 33). Lancet 352(9131) 837–853. https //doi.org/10.1016/S0140-6736(98)07019-6

66. Holman RR, Paul SK, Bethel MA, Matthews DR, Neil HA. 10-year follow-up of intensive glucose control in type 2 diabetes. *N Engl J Med.* 2008 Oct 9;359(15):1577-89. doi: 10.1056/NEJMoa0806470.

67. Gæde, P, Oellgaard, J, Carstensen, B., et al. Years of life gained by multifactorial intervention in patients with type 2 diabetes mellitus and microalbuminuria 21 years follow-up on the Steno-2 randomised trial. Diabetologia, 2006; 59(11), 2298–2307. https //doi.org/10.1007/s00125-016-4065-6

68. Folz, R., Laiteerapong, N. The legacy effect in diabetes are there long-term benefits. Diabetologia. 2021; 64, 2131–2137. https //doi.org/10.1007/s00125-021-05539-8

69. Wing RR, Egan C, Bahnson JL, et al., for the Look AHEAD Research Group. Long-term effects of a lifestyle intervention on weight and cardiovascular risk factors in individuals with type 2 diabetes mellitus four-year results of the Look AHEAD trial. *Arch Intern Med* 2010;170

70. Salvia MG. The Look AHEAD Trial: Translating Lessons Learned Into Clinical Practice and Further Study. Diabetes Spectr. 2017 Aug;30(3):166-170. doi: 10.2337/ds17-0016.

71. Salas-Salvadó J, Bulló M, Babio N, Martínez-González MÁ et al. Reduction in the incidence of type 2 diabetes with the Mediterranean diet Results of the PREDIMED-Reus nutrition intervention randomized trial. *Diabetes Care.* 2011;34 14–9.

72. Emilio Ros, Miguel A. Martínez-González, et al. Mediterranean Diet and Cardiovascular Health Teachings of the PREDIMED Study, Advances in Nutrition, Volume 5, Issue 3, May 2014, Pages 330S–336S, https //doi.org/10.3945/an.113.005389

73. Alison B. Evert, Michelle Dennison, Christopher D. Gardner, W. Timothy Garvey, et al. Nutrition Therapy for Adults With Diabetes or Prediabetes A Consensus Report. *Diabetes Care* 1 May 2019; 42 (5) 731–754. https //doi.org/10.2337/dci19-0014

74. Gang Hu, Cinzia Sarti, Pekka Jousilahti, Markku Peltonen, Qing Qiao. The Impact of History of Hypertension and Type 2 Diabetes at Baseline

on the Incidence of Stroke and Stroke Mortality. *Stroke* Volume 36, Issue 12, 1 December 2005; Pages 2538-2543
75. Meg G. Salvia; The Look AHEAD Trial Translating Lessons Learned Into Clinical Practice and Further Study. *Diabetes Spectr* 1 August 2017; 30 (3) 166–170. https //doi.org/10.2337/ds17-0016
76. Folz R, Laiteerapong N. The legacy effect in diabetes: are there long-term benefits? Diabetologia. 2021 Oct;64(10):2131-2137. doi: 10.1007/s00125-021-05539-8

Chapter 5

77. Kübler-Ross E. (1969). *On death and dying*. New York, NY: Macmillan.
78. Sevild CH, Niemiec CP, Bru LE, Dyrstad SM, Husebø AML. Initiation and maintenance of lifestyle changes among participants in a healthy life centre: a qualitative study. *BMC Public Health*. 2020 Jun 26;20(1):1006
79. Schmidt SK, Hemmestad L, MacDonald CS, Langberg H, Valentiner LS. Motivation and Barriers to Maintaining Lifestyle Changes in Patients with Type 2 Diabetes after an Intensive Lifestyle Intervention (The U-TURN Trial): A Longitudinal Qualitative Study. *Int J Environ Res Public Health*. 2020 Oct 13;17(20):7454
80. Koziol LF, Lutz JT. From movement to thought: the development of executive function. Appl Neuropsychol Child. 2013;2(2):104-15.
81. Shaffer J. Neuroplasticity and Clinical Practice: Building Brain Power for Health. *Front Psychol*. 2016 Jul 26;7:1118
82. Niazi AK, Niazi SK. Mindfulness-based stress reduction: a non-pharmacological approach for chronic illnesses. *N Am J Med Sci*. 2011 Jan;3(1):20-3.
83. Miller CK. Mindful Eating With Diabetes. *Diabetes Spectr*. 2017 May;30(2):89-94. doi: 10.2337/ds16-0039.
84. Holt, S. H., Miller, J. C., Petocz, P., & Farmakalidis, E. (1995). A satiety index of common foods. *Eur J Clin Nutr*, 49(9), 675-690

Chapter 6

85. Monteiro CA, Cannon G, Maubarac JC, et al. The UN decade of nutrition, the NOVA food classification, and the trouble with ultra-processing. *Public Health Nutr.* 2018;21(1):5-17
86. Monteiro CA, Cannon G, Levy RB, et al.. Ultra-processed foods: what they are and how to identify them. *Public Health Nutr.* 2019;22(5):936-941. DOI: 10.1017/S1368980018003762
87. Matos RA, Adams M, Sabaté J. Review: The Consumption of Ultra-Processed Foods and Non-communicable Diseases in Latin America. *Front Nutr.* 2021 Mar 24; 8:622714.
88. Marino M, Puppo F, Del Bo' C, Vinelli V, Riso P, Porrini M, Martini D. A Systematic Review of Worldwide Consumption of Ultra-Processed Foods: Findings and Criticisms. Nutrients. 2021 Aug 13;13(8):2778. doi: 10.3390/nu13082778.
89. Srour B, Fezeu LK, Kesse-Guyot E, Allès B, Debras C, et al. Ultraprocessed Food Consumption and Risk of Type 2 Diabetes Among Participants of the NutriNet-Santé Prospective Cohort. *JAMA Intern Med.* 2019 Dec 16;
90. Mendonça RD, Pimenta AM, Gea A, de la Fuente-Arrillaga C, Martinez-Gonzalez MA, Lopes AC, Bes-Rastrollo M. Ultraprocessed food consumption and risk of overweight and obesity: the University of Navarra Follow-Up (SUN) cohort study. Am J Clin Nutr. 2016 Nov;104(5):1433-1440. doi: 10.3945/ajcn.116.135004.
91. Matos RA, Adams M, Sabaté J. Review: The Consumption of Ultra-Processed Foods and Non-communicable Diseases in Latin America. *Front Nutr.* 2021 Mar 24; 8:622714.
92. Rico-CampÁ A, MartÁnez-GonzÁ¡lez M A, Alvarez-Alvarez I, et al. Association between consumption of ultra-processed foods and all cause mortality: SUN prospective cohort study *BMJ* 2019; 365 :l1949 doi:10.1136/bmj.l1949
93. Srour B, Fezeu LK, Kesse-Guyot E, et al. Ultraprocessed Food Consumption and Risk of Type 2 Diabetes Among Participants

of the NutriNet-Santé Prospective Cohort. *JAMA Intern Med.* 2020;180(2):283–291. doi:10.1001/jamainternmed.2019.5942

94. Advances in Food and Nutrition Research, Fidel Toldra, Characterization of the Degree of Food Processing in Relation With Its Health Potential and Effects. Anthony Fardet1- Academic Press, Elsevier, 2018.

95. Holt, S. H., & Miller, J. B. Particle size, satiety, and the glycaemic response. European Journal of Clinical Nutrition, 1994; 48(7), 496–502.

96. McRae MP. Health Benefits of Dietary Whole Grains: An Umbrella Review of Meta-analyses. *J Chiropr Med.* 2017 Mar;16(1):10-18. doi: 10.1016/j.jcm.2016.08.008. Epub 2016 Nov 18.

97. Anne Moorhead, S, Welch, R. W., Barbara, M., Livingstone, E., et al. The effects of the fibre content and physical structure of carrots on satiety and subsequent intakes when eaten as part of a mixed meal. The British journal of nutrition, 2006; 96(3), 587–595.

98. Ursell, L.K. et al. Defining the Human Microbiome. *Nutr Rev.* 2012 Aug; 70(Suppl 1): S38–S44.

99. Tsalamandris S, Antonopoulos A.S, Oikonomou E. et al. The role of inflammation in diabetes: Current concepts and future perspectives. *Eur. Cardiol. Rev.* 2019;14:50–59.

100. Payne AN, Chassard C, Lacroix C. Gut microbial adaptation to dietary consumption of fructose, artificial sweeteners and sugar alcohols: implications for host-microbe interactions contributing to obesity. *Obesity Rev.* 2012;13(9):799–809.

101. Furman, D., Campisi, J., Verdin, E. et al. Chronic inflammation in the etiology of disease across the life span. *Nat Med* 25, 1822–1832 (2019). https://doi.org/10.1038/s41591-019-0675-0

102. Neuenschwander M, Ballon A, Weber K S, Norat T, Aune D, Schwingshackl L et al. Role of diet in type 2 diabetes incidence: umbrella review of meta-analyses of prospective observational studies. *BMJ* 2019; 366 :l2368 doi:10.1136/bmj.l2368

103. Sørensen, L. B., Møller, P., Flint, A., Martens, M., & Raben, A. Effect of sensory perception of foods on appetite and food intake: a review of studies on humans. International journal of obesity and related

metabolic disorders: *journal of the International Association for the Study of Obesity*, 2003; 27(10), 1152–1166.

104. Dtnext: Why do your mothers' meals taste so good? https://www.dtnext.in/lifestyletopnews/2016/12/12/why-do-your-mothers-meals-taste-so-goodhttps://www.dtnext.in/lifestyletopnews/2016/12/12/why-do-your-mothers-meals-taste-so-good

105. Euromonitor International's2011 Annual Study of global consumers. Home Cooking and Eating Habits: Global Survey Analysis. http://blog.euromonitor.com/2012/04/home-cooking-and-eating-habits-global-survey-strategic-analysis.htm

106. Mills S, Brown H, Wieden W, White M, Adams J. Frequency of eating home-cooked meals and potential benefits for diet and health: a cross-sectional analysis of a population-based cohort study. *Int J Behav Nutr Phys Act*. 2017;14(1):109.

107. Julia A Wolfson, Sara N Bleich. Is cooking at home associated with better diet quality or weight-loss intention? *Public Health Nutrition*, 2014;

108. Katherine L. Hanna and Peter F. Collins, Relationship between living alone and food and nutrient intake. *Nutrition Reviews*, Volume 73, Issue 9, September 2015, Pages 594–611, https://doi.org/10.1093/nutrit/nuv02

109. Zong G, Eisenberg DM, Hu FB, Sun Q. Consumption of meals prepared at home and risk of type 2 diabetes: an analysis of two prospective cohort studies. *PLoS Med*. 2016;13(7):e1002052

110. Time: Homemade Meals Lower Risk of Diabetes, Study Says. https://time.com/4104061/homemade-meals-diabetes/

111. Dasgupta, K., Hajna, S., Joseph, L. et al. Effects of meal preparation training on body weight, glycemia, and blood pressure: results of a phase 2 trial in type 2 diabetes. Int J Behav Nutr Phys Act.2012; 9, 125 . https://doi.org/10.1186/1479-5868-9-125

Chapter 7

112. Hamdy O, Barakatun-Nisak MY. Nutrition in Diabetes. Endocrinol Metab Clin North Am. 2016 Dec;45(4):799-817. doi: 10.1016/j.ecl.2016.06.010.
113. American Diabetes Association Screening for type 2 diabetes. *Diabetes Care* 2004; 28 (Suppl. 1): S11– S14.
114. ElSayed NA, Aleppo G, Aroda VR, et al. 6. Glycemic Targets: Standards of Care in Diabetes-2023. *Diabetes Care* 2023; 46:S97.
115. Wei N, Zheng H, Nathan DM. Empirically establishing blood glucose targets to achieve HbA1c goals. *Diabetes Care* 2014; 37:1048.
116. Farahmand, M., Tehrani, F.R., Amiri, P. et al. Barriers to healthy nutrition: perceptions and experiences of Iranian women. *BMC Public Health* 12, 1064 (2012). https://doi.org/10.1186/1471-2458-12-1064
117. U.S. Department of Agriculture and U.S. Department of Health and Human Services. Dietary Guidelines for Americans, 2020-2025. (accessed on Jan 2023 https://www.dietaryguidelines.gov/)
118. Blonde L, Umpierrez GE, Reddy SS, et al. American Association of Clinical Endocrinology Clinical Practice Guideline: Developing a Diabetes Mellitus Comprehensive Care Plan-2022 Update. Endocr Pract. 2022 Oct;28(10):923-1049. doi: 10.1016/j.eprac.2022.08.002.
119. Lebovitz HE, Austin MM, Blonde L, Davidson JA, Del Prato S, Gavin JR, Handelsman Y, Jellinger PS, Levy P, Riddle MC, Roberts VL, Siminerio LM: ACE/AACE Consensus Conference on the implementation of outpatient management of diabetes mellitus: consensus conference recommendations. *Endocr Pract* 2006; 12 (Suppl. 1): 6– 12
120. American Diabetes Association Professional Practice Committee; 6. Glycemic Targets: *Standards of Medical Care in Diabetes—2022*. *Diabetes Care* 1 January 2022; 45 (Supplement_1): S83–S96. https://doi.org/10.2337/dc22-S006
121. NICE (2015) Type 2 diabetes in adults: management [NG28]. NICE, London. Available at: www.nice.org.uk/guidance/ng28

122. Gaede P, Lund-Andersen H, Parving HH, Pedersen O. Effect of a multifactorial intervention on mortality in type 2 diabetes. *N Engl J Med* 2008;358:580–591

123. International Diabetes Federation: Guideline for the management of postmeal glucose, Brussels, IDF:1–27, 2007. Available from www.idf.org.

124. Lebovitz HE, Austin MM, Blonde L, et al. ACE/AACE Consensus Conference on the implementation of outpatient management of diabetes mellitus: consensus conference recommendations. *Endocr Pract* 2006; 12 (Suppl. 1): 6– 12

125. NICE (2015) Type 2 diabetes in adults: management [NG28]. NICE, London. Available at: www.nice.org.uk/guidance/ng28

126. Whitton C, Ramos-García C, Kirkpatrick SI, et al. A Systematic Review Examining Contributors to Misestimation of Food and Beverage Intake Based on Short-Term Self-Report Dietary Assessment Instruments Administered to Adults. *Adv Nutr*. 2022 Dec 22;13(6):2620-2665. doi: 10.1093/advances/nmac085.

127. Almiron-Roig, E., Solis-Trapala, I., Dodd, J., & Jebb, S. A. Estimating food portions. Influence of unit number, meal type and energy density. *Appetite*, 2013; 71, 95–103. https://doi.org/10.1016/j.appet.2013.07.012

128. Thompson, S.V., Winham, D.M. & Hutchins, A.M. Bean and rice meals reduce postprandial glycemic response in adults with type 2 diabetes: a cross-over study. *Nutr J* 11, 23 (2012

129. Sun L, Ranawana DV, Leow MK, Henry CJ. Effect of chicken, fat and vegetable on glycaemia and insulinaemia to a white rice-based meal in healthy adults. *Eur J Nutr*. 2014 Dec;53(8):1719-26

130. A. Josse, C. Kendall, L. Augustin, P. Ellis, D. Jenkins Almonds and post-prandial glycemia—a dose-response study. *Metabolism*, 56 (2007), pp. 400-404.

131. Ostman E, Granfeldt Y, Persson L, Björck I. Vinegar supplementation lowers glucose and insulin responses and increases satiety after a bread meal in healthy subjects. *Eur J Clin Nutr*. 2005 Sep;59(9):983-8. doi: 10.1038/sj.ejcn.1602197. PMID: 16015276.

132. Lutgarda Bozzetto, Antonio Alderisio, Marisa Giorgini, et al. Extra-Virgin Olive Oil Reduces Glycemic Response to a High–Glycemic Index Meal in Patients With Type 1 Diabetes: A Randomized Controlled Trial. *Diabetes Care* 1 April 2016; 39 (4): 518–524
133. Alpana P. Shukla, Radu G. Iliescu, Catherine E. Thomas, Louis J. Aronne; Food Order Has a Significant Impact on Postprandial Glucose and Insulin Levels. *Diabetes Care* 1 July 2015; 38 (7)
134. Li Z, Hu Y, Yan R, et al. Twenty Minute Moderate-Intensity Post-Dinner Exercise Reduces the Postprandial Glucose Response in Chinese Patients with Type 2 Diabetes. Med Sci Monit. 2018 Oct 8;24:7170-7177. doi: 10.12659/MSM.910827.
135. Haxhi J, Scotto di Palumbo A, Sacchetti M. Exercising for metabolic control: is timing important? *Ann Nutr Metab* (2013) 62(1):14–25
136. Daenen S, Sola-Gazagnes A, M'Bemba J, et al. Peak-time determination of post-meal glucose excursions in insulin-treated diabetic patients. Diabetes Metab (2010) 36(2):165–9
137. Erickson ML, Little JP, Gay JL, McCully KK, Jenkins NT. Postmeal exercise blunts postprandial glucose excursions in people on metformin monotherapy. *J Appl Physiol* (1985) (2017) 123(3):444–50
138. Gray A, Threlkeld RJ. Nutritional Recommendations for Individuals with Diabetes. [Updated 2019 Oct 13]. In: Feingold KR, Anawalt B, Blackman MR, et al., editors. Endotext [Internet]. South Dartmouth (MA): MDText.com, Inc.; 2000-. Available from: https://www.ncbi.nlm.nih.gov/books/NBK279012/
139. https://www.fda.gov/food/consumers/advice-about-eating-fish
140. Rehman A, Saeed A, Kanwal R, Ahmad S, Changazi SH. Therapeutic Effect of Sunflower Seeds and Flax Seeds on Diabetes. *Cureus*. 2021 Aug 17;13(8):e17256. doi: 10.7759/cureus.17256.
141. Vuksan V, Choleva L, Jovanovski E, et al. Comparison of flax (Linum usitatissimum) and Salba-chia (Salvia hispanica L.) seeds on postprandial glycemia and satiety in healthy individuals: a randomized, controlled, crossover study. *Eur J Clin Nutr.* 2017 Feb;71(2):234-238. doi: 10.1038/ejcn.2016.148.

142. Alwosais EZM, Al-Ozairi E, Zafar TA, Alkandari S. Chia seed (Salvia hispanica L.) supplementation to the diet of adults with type 2 diabetes improved systolic blood pressure: A randomized controlled trial. *Nutrition and Health*. 2021;27(2):181-189. doi:10.1177/0260106020981819

143. Carlsen, M.H., Halvorsen, B.L., Holte, K. et al. The total antioxidant content of more than 3100 foods, beverages, spices, herbs and supplements used worldwide. *Nutr J* 9, 3 (2010).

144. Rogers PJ, Hohoff C, Heatherley SV, et al. Association of the anxiogenic and alerting effects of caffeine with ADORA2A and ADORA1 polymorphisms and habitual level of caffeine consumption. *Neuropsychopharmacology*, 2010, 35(9), 1973-1983 | added to CENTRAL: 31 January 2011 | 2011 Issue 1
Ding M, Bhupathiraju SN, Chen M, van Dam RM, Hu FB. Caffeinated and decaffeinated coffee consumption and risk of type 2 diabetes: a systematic review and a dose-response meta-analysis. *Diabetes Care*. 2014 Feb;37(2):569-86

145. Ding M, Bhupathiraju SN, Chen M, van Dam RM, Hu FB. Caffeinated and decaffeinated coffee consumption and risk of type 2 diabetes: a systematic review and a dose-response meta-analysis. *Diabetes Care*. 2014 Feb;37(2):569-86.

146. Poole R, Kennedy OJ, Roderick P, et al.. Coffee consumption and health: umbrella review of meta-analyses of multiple health outcomes. *BMJ*. 2017 Nov 22;359:j5024. doi: 10.1136/bmj.j5024.

147. Bonuccelli G, Sotgia F, Lisanti MP. Matcha green tea (MGT) inhibits the propagation of cancer stem cells (CSCs), by targeting mitochondrial metabolism, glycolysis and multiple cell signalling pathways. *Aging (Albany NY)*. 2018 Aug 23;10(8):1867-1883.

148. Yi M, Wu X, Zhuang W, et al. Tea Consumption and Health Outcomes: Umbrella Review of Meta-Analyses of Observational Studies in Humans. *Mol Nutr Food Res*. 2019 Aug;63(16):e1900389. doi: 10.1002/mnfr.201900389.

149. Rusak G, Komes D, Likić S, Horžić D, Kovač M. Phenolic content and antioxidative capacity of green and white tea extracts depending

on extraction conditions and the solvent used. *Food Chem.* 2008 Oct 15;110(4):852-8.
150. Deng R. A review of the hypoglycemic effects of five commonly used herbal food supplements. *Recent Pat Food Nutr Agric.* 2012 Apr 1;4(1):50-60. doi: 10.2174/2212798411204010050.
151. Akhtar A S, Ramzan A, Ali A, Ahmad M. Effect of Amla fruit (Emblica officinalis Gaertn.) on blood glucose and lipid profile of normal subjects and type 2 diabetic patients. *International Journal of Food Sciences and Nutrition*, 2011;62:6, 609-616, DOI: 10.3109/09637486.2011.560565
152. Deng R. A review of the hypoglycemic effects of five commonly used herbal food supplements. *Recent Pat Food Nutr Agric.* 2012 Apr 1;4(1):50-60
153. Hassani SS, Fallahi Arezodar F, Esmaeili SS, Gholami-Fesharaki M. Effect of Fenugreek Use on Fasting Blood Glucose, Glycosylated Hemoglobin, Body Mass Index, Waist Circumference, Blood Pressure and Quality of Life in Patients with Type 2 Diabetes Mellitus: A Randomized, Double-Blinded, Placebo-Controlled Clinical Trials. *Galen Med J.* 2019 Mar 30;8:e1432. doi: 10.31661/gmj.v8i0.1432.
154. Madar Z, Abel R, Samish S, Arad J. Glucose-lowering effect of fenugreek in non-insulin-dependent diabetics. Eur J Clin Nutr. 1988 Jan;42(1):51-4. PMID: 3286242.
155. Diabetes.co.uk: Fenugreek and Diabetes. https://www.diabetes.co.uk/natural-therapies/fenugreek.html
156. Neelakantan, N., Narayanan, M., de Souza, R.J. et al. Effect of fenugreek (Trigonella foenum-graecumL.) intake on glycemia: a meta-analysis of clinical trials. *Nutr J* 13, 7 (2014). https://doi.org/10.1186/1475-2891-13-7
157. Owen RW, Mier W, Giacosa A, et al. Phenolic compounds and squalene in olive oils: the concentration and antioxidant potential of total phenols, simple phenols, secoiridoids, lignansand squalene. *Food Chem Toxicol* 2000; 38: 647–659
158. Lutgarda Bozzetto L, Antonio Alderisio A, Marisa Giorgini M, et al. Extra-Virgin Olive Oil Reduces Glycemic Response to a High–Glycemic Index Meal in Patients With Type 1 Diabetes: A Randomized

Controlled Trial. *Diabetes Care* 1 April 2016; 39 (4): 518–524. https://doi.org/10.2337/dc15-2189

159. Schwingshackl L, Lampousi AM, Portillo MP, et al. Olive oil in the prevention and management of type 2 diabetes mellitus: a systematic review and meta-analysis of cohort studies and intervention trials. Nutr Diabetes. 2017 Apr 10;7(4):e262. doi: 10.1038/nutd.2017.12.

160. Pauline, J., and Maddox. Cinnamon in the Treatment of Type II Diabetes. *J. Interdiscip. Graduate Res.* 2017; 2 (1).

161. Santos, H. O., and da Silva, G. A. R. To what Extent Does Cinnamon Administration Improve the Glycemic and Lipid Profiles? *Clin. Nutr.* 2018; ESPEN 27, 1–9. doi:10.1016/j.clnesp.2018.07.011

162. Abraham, K., Wöhrlin, F., Lindtner, O., Heinemeyer, G., and Lampen, A. Toxicology and Risk Assessment of Coumarin: Focus on Human. Data. Mol. *Nutr. Food Res.*2010; 54 (2), 228–239. doi:10.1002/mnfr.200900281

163. Hossein, N. . Effect of Cinnamon Zeylanicum Essence and Distillate on the Clotting Time. *J. Med. Plant Res.* 2013; 7 (17), 1339–1343.

164. Khan A, Safdar M, Ali Khan MM, Khattak KN, Anderson RA. Cinnamon improves the glucose and lipids of people with type 2 diabetes. *Diabetes Care.* 2003 Dec;26(12):3215-8. doi: 10.2337/diacare.26.12.3215. PMID: 14633804.

165. Griffin Morgan. Nov 6, 2022, Cinnamon. https://www.webmd.com/diet/supplement-guide-cinnamon. (Accessed on Jan 26, 2023.)

166. Pauline, J., and Maddox. Cinnamon in the Treatment of Type II Diabetes. *J. Interdiscip. Graduate Res.* 2017;2 (1).

Chapter 8

167. Sheri R. Colberg, Ronald J. Sigal, Jane E. Yardley, et al. Physical Activity/Exercise and Diabetes: A Position Statement of the American Diabetes Association. *Diabetes Care* 1 November 2016; 39 (11): 2065–2079. https://doi.org/10.2337/dc16-1728

168. Lee, I. M., Shiroma, E. J., Lobelo, F., Puska, P., Blair, S. N., Katzmarzyk, P. T., & Lancet Physical Activity Series Working Group. Effect of

physical inactivity on major non-communicable diseases worldwide: an analysis of burden of disease and life expectancy. *Lancet* (London, England), 2012;380(9838), 219–229. https://doi.org/10.1016/S0140-6736(12)61031-9

169. Jonas S, Phillips EM. Exercise is Medicine: A clinician's guide to Exercise prescription. Philadelphia, PA: Lippincott Williams & Wilkins; 2009:101.

170. Sangwung, P., Petersen, K. F., Shulman, G. I., & Knowles, J. W. Mitochondrial Dysfunction, Insulin Resistance, and Potential Genetic Implications. Endocrinology, 2020; 161(4), bqaa017. https://doi.org/10.1210/endocr/bqaa017

171. Jitrapakdee S, Wutthisathapornchai A, Wallace JC, MacDonald MJ. Regulation of insulin secretion: role of mitochondrial signalling. Diabetologia. 2010 Jun;53(6):1019-32. doi: 10.1007/s00125-010-1685-0.

172. Schrauwen, P., van Marken Lichtenbelt, W.D. Combatting type 2 diabetes by turning up the heat. *Diabetologia* 59, 2269–2279 (2016). https://doi.org/10.1007/s00125-016-4068-3

173. Richter EA, Hargreaves M. Exercise, GLUT4, and skeletal muscle glucose uptake. *Physiol Rev.* 2013 Jul;93(3):993-1017. doi: 10.1152/physrev.00038.2012.

175. Ljubičić M, Matek Sarić M, Klarin I, Rumbak I, et al. Emotions and Food Consumption: Emotional Eating Behavior in a European Population. *Foods.* 2023 Feb 17;12(4):872. doi: 10.3390/foods12040872.

176. Diabetes A to Z: what you need to know about diabetes, simply put. American Diabetes Association.7th Edition, 2015.

177. Gordon BA, Bird SR, MacIsaac RJ, Benson AC. Does a single bout of resistance or aerobic exercise after insulin dose reduction modulate glycaemic control in type 2 diabetes? A randomised cross-over trial. *J Sci Med Sport.* 2016 Oct;19(10):795-9. doi: 10.1016/j.jsams.2016.01.004.

178. Dempsey PC, Owen N, Biddle SJ, Dunstan DW. Managing sedentary behavior to reduce the risk of diabetes and cardiovascular disease. *Curr Diab Rep* 2014;14:522

179. Jiménez-Maldonado A, García-Suárez PC, Rentería I, Moncada-Jiménez J, Plaisance EP. Impact of high-intensity interval training and sprint interval training on peripheral markers of glycemic control in metabolic syndrome and type 2 diabetes. Biochim Biophys Acta Mol Basis Dis. 2020 Aug 1;1866(8):165820. doi: 10.1016/j.bbadis.2020.165820.
180. Chen, Z., Ye, X., Xia, Y., et al . Effect of Pilates on Glucose and Lipids: A Systematic Review and Meta-Analysis of Randomized Controlled Trials. *Frontiers in physiology*, 2021; 12, 641968. https://doi.org/10.3389/fphys.2021.641968
181. Turner, G., Quigg, S., Davoren, P. et al. Resources to Guide Exercise Specialists Managing Adults with Diabetes. *Sports Med - Open* 5, 20 (2019). https://doi.org/10.1186/s40798-019-0192-1
182. Magkos F, Tsekouras Y, Kavouras SA, Mittendorfer B, Sidossis LS. Improved insulin sensitivity after a single bout of exercise is curvilinearly related to exercise energy expenditure. *Clin Sci* (Lond) 2008;114:59–64.
183. Sargent, C., Zhou, X., Matthews, R. W., et al. Daily Rhythms of Hunger and Satiety in Healthy Men during One Week of Sleep Restriction and Circadian Misalignment. *International journal of environmental research and public health*, 2016;13(2), 170. https://doi.org/10.3390/ijerph13020170.
184. Zhilei Shan, Hongfei Ma, Manling Xie, et al. Sleep Duration and Risk of Type 2 Diabetes: A Meta-analysis of Prospective Studies. *Diabetes Care* 1 March 2015; 38 (3): 529–537. https://doi.org/10.2337/dc14-2073
185. Boden G, Chen X, Urbain JL (1996) Evidence for a circadian rhythm of insulin sensitivity in patients with NIDDM caused by cyclic changes in hepatic glucose production. Diabetes 45(8):1044–1050. https://doi.org/10.2337/diab.45.8.1044
186. A.D.A.M. Medical Encyclopedia. (2020, April 9). Changing your sleep habits. MedlinePlus. Retrieved May 14, 2022, from https://medlineplus.gov/ency/patientinstructions/000757.htm
187. Binks, H., E Vincent, G., Gupta, C., Irwin, C., & Khalesi, S. (2020). Effects of diet on sleep: A narrative review. Nutrients, 12(4), 936. https://pubmed.ncbi.nlm.nih.gov/32230944/

188. Aikens JE. Prospective associations between emotional distress and poor outcomes in type 2 diabetes. *Diabetes Care*; 2012;35:2472–2478
189. Brinkhues S, Dukers-Muijrers NHTM, Hoebe CJPA, et al. Social Network Characteristics Are Associated With Type 2 Diabetes Complications: The Maastricht Study. *Diabetes Care.* 2018 Aug;41(8):1654-1662. doi: 10.2337/dc17-2144.
190. Makhmur, S., Rath, S. PERMA Dimensions of Well-Being Among Diabetic and Non-Diabetic Adults: Evidence from Two Diabetic Care Hospitals in Odisha. *Psychol Stud*; 2022. 67, 468–479. https://doi.org/10.1007/s12646-022-00677-4
191. Aknin, L. B., Dunn, E. W., & Norton, M. I. Happiness runs in a circular motion: Evidence for a positive feedback loop between prosocial spending and happiness. *Journal of Happiness Studies*; 2012.13(2), 347-355.
192. Yi-Frazier, J., Hilliard, M., Cochrane, K. & Hood, K. The Impact of Positive Psychology on Diabetes Outcomes: A Review. *Psychology.* 2012. 3, 1116-1124. doi: 10.4236/psych.2012.312A165.
193. AlAmmar WA, Albeesh FH, Khattab RY. Food and Mood: the Correspondence Effect. *Curr Nutr Rep.* 2020 Sep;9(3):296-308. doi: 10.1007/s13668-020-00331-3.

Chapter 9

194. Makroum MA, Adda M, Bouzouane A, Ibrahim H. Machine Learning and Smart Devices for Diabetes Management: *Systematic Review.* Sensors (Basel). 2022 Feb 25;22(5):1843.
195. Victoria Millson, Peter Hammond, June 2020, How to analyse CGM data: A structured and practical approach. https://diabetesonthenet.com/journal-diabetes-nursing/how-analyse-cgm-data-structured-and-practical-approach/(accessed jan, 2023)
196. Fleming GA, Petrie JR, Bergenstal RM, et al. Diabetes Digital App Technology: Benefits, Challenges, and Recommendations. A Consensus Report by the European Association for the Study of Diabetes (EASD) and the American Diabetes Association (ADA) Diabetes G. Diabetes

Technology Working Group. *Diabetes Care* 1 January 2020; 43 (1): 250–260.

197. Wang Y., Wu X., Mo X. A novel adaptive-weighted-average framework for blood glucose prediction. *Diabetes Technol. Ther.* 2013;15:792–801. doi: 10.1089/dia.2013.0104.

198. Berget C, Messer LH, Forlenza GP. A Clinical Overview of Insulin Pump Therapy for the Management of Diabetes: Past, Present, and Future of Intensive Therapy. *Diabetes Spectr.* 2019 Aug;32(3):194-204. doi: 10.2337/ds18-0091.

Appendix

199. American Diabetes Association Professional Practice Committee. 9. Pharmacologic approaches to glycemic treatment: Standards of medical care in diabetes—2022. Diabetes Care. 2022;45(Supplement_1):S125-S143. doi:10.2337/dc22-S009

200. Tso LO, Costello MF, Albuquerque LE et al. Metformin treatment before and during IVF or ICSI in women with polycystic ovary syndrome. Cochrane Database of Systematic Reviews. 2009, Issue 2. Art. No.: CD006105

201. McIntosh CH, Demuth HU, Pospisilik JA, Pederson R. "Dipeptidyl peptidase IV inhibitors: how do they work as new antidiabetic agents?". *Regulatory Peptides.* 2005; 128 (2): 159–65. doi:10.1016/j.regpep.2004.06.001

202. Saini, R., & Badole, S. L. Chapter 28 - Bioactive Compounds Increase Incretins with Beneficial Effects on Diabetes. Ronald Ross Watson, Betsy B. Dokken Eds. Glucose Intake and Utilization in Pre-Diabetes and Diabetes,
Academic Press,2015,Pages 349-353,ISBN 9780128000939, https://doi.org/10.1016/B978-0-12-800093-9.00028-4.

203. Shah, M., & Vella, A. Effects of GLP-1 on appetite and weight. Reviews in endocrine & metabolic disorders, 15(3), 2014; 181–187. https://doi.org/10.1007/s11154-014-9289-5

204. Ghani, U. (2019). Alpha-glucosidase Inhibitors: Clinically Promising Candidates for Anti-diabetic Drug Discovery. Netherlands: Elsevier Science.
205. Vaduganathan M, Docherty KF, Claggett BL, et al. Solomon SD. SGLT-2 inhibitors in patients with heart failure: a comprehensive meta-analysis of five randomised controlled trials. *Lancet*. 2022 Sep 3;400(10354):757-767.

INDEX

Note: Page numbers followed by f and t indicates figure and table respectively.

A

Absorption, 26–27
   cholesterol, 62
   fructose and galactose, 68
   glucose, 34–35
   vitamin B12, 297
Acarbose (Precose), 300
Active movement, 15–16, 232–233
   blood glucose, 235–236
   insulin action and, 243–244
ADA. *See* American Diabetes Association (ADA)
Adenosine triphosphate (ATP), 22, 68, 236
Adipose tissue, 23, 27
   fat storage in, 30
   inflammation, 28
   insulin resistance in, 29
Adrenaline, 247
Adult-onset diabetes. *See* Type 2 diabetes
Aerobic exercise, 238
ALA. *See* Alpha-linolenic acid (ALA)
Albumin-to creatinine ratio, 94
Alcohol abuse, 38. *See also* Pancreatitis
Alcohol intake, 256
Alpha-glucosidase inhibitors (AGIs), 300–301

Alpha-linolenic acid (ALA), 79
American Association of Clinical Endocrinologists, 207
American Diabetes Association (ADA)
   carbohydrates, 51, 246
   diagnostic criteria, 43, 43t
   fasting blood glucose, 207
   post-meal glucose, 184, 210
   pre-meal glucose, 184, 208
Amla, 221–222
Animal fat, 83
Antioxidant-rich foods, 217–218
Anxiety, 257–259
Appetite, 130–131
   stress and, 264
Apps, 274–275
Artificial Intelligence, 276
Atherosclerosis, 99
Atkins diet, 50
Autonomic neuropathy, 102

B

Balancing exercises, 239
Belief system, 119–120
   ask yourself, 122
   with facts and references, 122
   identify, 121–122
   positive, 122
   reinforcement of, 122–123

Index

Berries, 218–219
Beta cells (β-cells), 26
   dysfunction of, 31–32
   gestational diabetes, 36
   type 1 diabetes, 37
Black tea, 220
Blood glucose, 1, 6, 8, 11, 16, 90, 178
   active movement, 235–236
   diet, 14
   equilibrium, 33
   exercises, 244
   fasting, 44, 206–208
   flaxseeds, 216
   fresh fruits, 66
   gestational diabetes mellitus, 36
   high concentrations of, 91
   hypoglycaemia, 95
   insulin resistance, 24f–25f
   liver and insulin, 21
   post-meal, 44, 209–210
   prediabetes, 33
   pre-meal, 208
   sleep and, 214, 251–257
   stress management, 16, 258
   technology
      continuous glucose monitoring, 271–273
      glucometers, 270–271
   tracking, 180
   type 1 diabetes, 37
   ultra-processed foods, 155–157
Blood lipid levels, 8, 80, 235
Blood pressure, 1, 8, 235
   high, 92–93
   measurement, 277
   systolic, 92
BMI. *See* Body mass index (BMI)
Body mass index (BMI), 32
Body weight, 94
Boredom eating, 228
Brain health, 100–101
Bread, choosing, 64
Bright fruits, 222
Brown bread, 63

C

Caffeine, 219–220
Calorie, 199t–201t
   calculator, 198
   consumption of, 13
   overconsumption of, 28
Canagliflozin (Invokana), 301
Cancer, 10
   breast, 233
   colon, 233
   colorectal, 61
   lung, 93
   pancreatic, 57
Canned foods, 146
Carbohydrates, 2
   complex, 53–57
   dietary, 49–53
   digestion and, 67–70
   food groups, 191
   fruit and vegetable, 65–66
   grains, 58
   hidden sources of, 192
   metabolism of, 69
   milk, 66–67
   quality of, 51, 203, 212
   quantity of, 51, 203
   refined, 57–58
   simple, 53–57
   structure of, 52
      pyramid of, 56f
   unrefined, 57–58
Cardiovascular disease (CVD), 1, 109
Cataracts, 101–102
CBT. *See* Cognitive behavioural therapy (CBT)
Cellulose, 56

CGM. *See* Continuous glucose monitoring (CGM)
Chemical-induced diabetes, 38
Chia seeds, 217
Cholesterol, 94
Chronic kidney disease, 10
Chronic stress, 258, 267
Cinnamon, 225
Circadian rhythms, 252
   natural light, 255
   type 2 diabetes, 253–254
Coffee, 219–221
Cognitive behavioural therapy (CBT), 16, 260–262
Compensation skills, 229
Complex carbohydrates, 53–57, 191
   chemical structures, 54
   food label for
      darker, do not assume, 62–63
      ingredients list, 63–65
      package, 62
   grains and beans, 56
Conditioning, 12–13
   belief system, 119–123
   decision, 117–119
   defined, 113
   emotions, 123–124
   mindful eating, 124–141
   motivation, 114–117
Continuous glucose monitoring (CGM), 225–227
   device, 271–273
Coronary artery disease, 10
Cortisol, 264
C-peptide, 46
C-reactive protein (CRP), 61, 162
CRP. *See* C-reactive protein (CRP)
Culinary medicine, 169

D

Dapagliflozin (Farxiga), 301
Dark chocolate, 222–223
Dawn phenomenon, 248, 253
Decision, 117–119
Dental problems, 103
Depression, 39
Diabetes, 1, 4, 17, 90–91, 113. *See also* Type 1 diabetes; Type 2 diabetes
   acute complications of
      diabetic ketoacidosis, 97–98
      hypoglycaemia, 95–97
   chronic complications of, 98–99
   as chronic disease, 7
   complications of, 92, 95
      Diabetes Control and Complications Trial, 104–105
      gums, 103
      landmark clinical trials in, 104
      legacy effect, 107, 109–110
      Look AHEAD trial, 108
      PREDIMED study, 108–109
      skin, 103
      Steno-2 trial, 106–107
      teeth, 103
      United Kingdom Prospective Diabetes Study, 105–106
   counseling, 7
   diagnosis of, 3, 5, 6
      criteria for, 43t
      tests, 42
   during pregnancy, 2
   early signs of, 39
   hyperglycemia, 11
   macrovascular complications of
      brain health, 100–101
      heart health, 99–100
      lower limbs, 101
   microvascular complications of
      eye health, 101–102
      kidney health, 102–103
      nerve health, 102

with obesity, 32–33
prevalence of, 13
reversed, 44–45
technology
  apps, 274–275
  fitness trackers, 275–276
  insulin pump therapy, 279–281
  smart insulin pens, 278–279
  smart watches, 276–277
types of, 33
  gestational diabetes mellitus, 36–37
  prediabetes, 33–34
  type 1, 37–38
  type 2, 35–36, 35f
Diabetes Control and Complications Trial (DCCT), 104–105
Diabetic ketoacidosis (DKA), 97–98
Diabetic kidney disease, 103
Diabetic nephropathy, 103
Dialysis, 90
Dietary carbohydrates, 49–53
  categories of, 55t
  composition of, 50
Dietary cholesterol, 83–84
  excessive, consuming, 84–86
  in food items, 83t
Dietary fats, 73–75
Dietary fibre, 193, 212
Digestion, 300
  carbohydrates and, 67–70
  food matrix in, 54f
Digestive enzymes, 66
Dipeptidyl peptidase-4 inhibitors (DPP-4) inhibitors, 298
Disaccharides, 52
DKA. *See* Diabetic ketoacidosis (DKA)
Docosahexaenoic acid (DHA), 79

Dual therapy, 297–298
Dulaglutide (Trulicity), 300
Dysbiosis, 160
Dyslipidemia, 94

E

Eating, 119, 154, 201. *See also* Mindful eating
  emotional, 137
  healthy, 15, 204
Ectopic fat, 28
Eicosapentaenoic acid (EPA), 79
Emotional eating, 137
Emotions, 123–124
Empagliflozin (Jardiance), 301
Endorphins, 222, 264
Epidemiology of Diabetes Interventions and Complications (EDIC), 105
Ertugliflozin (Steglatro), 301
Exenatide (Byetta), 300
Exenatide Extended-Release (Bydureon), 300
Exercises, 15, 232–233
  after, 249
    eat, 249–250
    inject insulin, 250–251
  baseline activity level, 240
  before, 244
    eat, 247
    inject insulin, 245–246
    oral medications, 245
    snack, 247
  blood glucose, 244
  during, 247–249
  fitness, 240–241
  glucose transporter channels, 236–237
  happy hormones and, 237
  intensity of, 240
  mitochondrial function and, 236
  150 minutes, 241–242

rule of thumb for, 241
stress, 265
types of, 238–239
Extra virgin olive oil, 224

F

FAO. *See* Food and Agriculture Organization (FAO)
Fast food, 148
Fasting blood glucose, 206–208
Fat cells, 27
Fatigue, 39
Fatty acids, 26–27, 29
    excessive, in liver, 78
    LDL cholesterol, 79
    omega-3, 79–80
    omega-6, 80
    protein transport, 30
    short-chain, 66
    unsaturated, 79
Fatty fish, 216
Fatty liver disease, 10, 78
Fatty meal, 27–29
Fenugreek, 223–224
Fibre, 56, 59, 66
    dietary, 193
    fenugreek, 223
    fruits and vegetables, 66
    insoluble, 66
    starches, 65
    whole grains, 61
Fibromyalgia, 39
15-15 Rule, 96–97
'Fight or flight' response, 258, 262
Fish, 216
Fitness, 240–241. *See also* Exercises
    trackers, 275–276
5C lifestyle prescription, 12
    active movement, 15–16, 231–267
    choose, cook and eat real food, 13–14, 143–173
    condition your mind, 12–13, 111–142
    meal planning, 14–15, 174–230
    relaxation, 231–267
    sound sleep, 15–16, 231–267
    stress management, 15–16
    technology, 16–17, 268–283
Flaxseeds, 216
Flexibility (stretching), 239
Food and Agriculture Organization (FAO), 50
Food and Drug Administration (FDA), 215
Food groups, 188–189, 189t–191t
Food labelling
    for complex carbohydrates
        darker, do not assume, 62–63
        ingredients list, 63–65
        package, 62
    laws, 62
Food matrix, in digestion/absorption, 54f
Food processing. *See* Processed foods
FPG. *See* Fasting plasma glucose (FPG)
Fructose, 21, 52, 68, 159–160, 204–205
Fruits, 65–66, 150t
    bright, 222
    juice, 204–206, 206t
Fullness, 131–132, 157, 163

G

Galactose, 21, 52, 68
GDM. *See* Gestational diabetes mellitus (GDM)
Gemigliptin (Zemiglo), 298
Genetic predisposition, 31
Gestational diabetes mellitus (GDM), 36–37
GI. *See* Glycemic index (GI)

GIP receptor, 300
GL. *See* Glycemic load (GL)
Glaucoma, 101–102
Gliflozins, 301
Glimepiride (amary), 302
Glipizide (Glucitrol), 302
Glitazones, 302
Glucagon, 298
Glucagon-like peptide (GLP-1)
  agonist, 298–299
Glucagon-like peptide (GLP-1)
  inhibitors, 299–300
Glucagon-like peptide (GLP-1)
  receptor agonists, 300
Glucometers, 181, 270–271
Gluconeogenesis, 68
Glucophage, 297
Glucose, 11, 52, 243
  absorption, 35
  control, 93
  as glycogen, 68
  insulin, 19
  lowering foods, 223
  post-meal, 184
  pre-meal, 184
  rate of uptake of, 67
  symptoms, 95
Glucose transporter channels,
  236–237
GLUT4 receptors, 237
Glyburide (Diabeta), 302
Glycated haemoglobin (HbA1C),
  42–43, 45, 93–94, 209, 225
Glycemic control, 36, 51, 93, 106,
  205, 216
Glycemic index (GI), 51, 70,
  189t–191t
  carbohydrates, 213
  factors, 71–72
  food, ripeness of, 71
  post-meal glucose response on,
    72f

virgin olive oil, 213
white rice, 212
whole grains, 71
Glycemic load (GL), 72–73
Glycogen, 26, 68
Grains, 1–2, 150t, 193, 197–198
  refined, 58–60, 59f
  whole, 58–60, 59f
Green tea, 220
Gum infections, 103
Gut health, 158–161

H
Haemorrhagic stroke, 100
HbA1C. *See* Glycated haemoglobin
  (HbA1C)
Health Professionals' Follow-Up
  Study, 81
Healthy eating, 192
Heart disease, 14, 57, 84–86
Heart health, 99–100
High-density lipoprotein (HDL)
  cholesterol, 85
High-intensity interval training
  (HIIT), 243
Home cooking, 168
Humulin N, 305–306
Hunger, 130, 157–158, 202
Hunger-fullness scale, 133t–134t
Hunger fullness tracker log, 134–
  135, 135t–136t
Hyperglycaemia, 98, 253
Hyperglycemia, 11, 30, 48
Hyperinsulinemia, 30
Hypertension, 1, 20, 102
  defined, 92
  excessive weight, 94
Hypoglycaemia, 95, 245, 250
  simple carbohydrates, 96
  in sleep, 97

I

IDF. *See* International Diabetes Federation (IDF)
Incretin mimetics, 298–299
Infections, 101
   gum, 103
   tooth, 103
Inflammation, 158, 161–162
   acute, 161–162
   chronic, 161–162
Insomnia, 16, 254
Insulin, 19, 69, 206, 237
   active movement and, 243–244
   after exercise, 250–251
   before exercise, 245–246
   diabetic ketoacidosis, 98
   excessive accumulation of, 30
   exogenous, 38
   as fat-storage hormone, 27
   functions of, 21
   onset, 303
   peak, 303
   premixed, 305–306
   pump therapy, 279–281
   secretagogues, 301–302
Insulin-dependent diabetes. *See* Type 1 diabetes
Insulin detemir, 305
Insulin glargine, 305
Insulin isophane, 305
Insulin Lispro, 306
Insulin resistance, 19, 28, 30, 258
   adipose tissue, consequences of, 29
   blood glucose spike, 24f–25f
   carbohydrate-rich meal, 21–23
   defined, 22
   genetic predisposition, 31
   gestational diabetes, 36
   human physiology, 20–21
   low-calorie diet, 76
   saturated fat, 76–77
   ultra-processed foods, 155–157
   unsaturated fats, 78
   weight gain, 44
Ipragliflozin (Suglat), 301
Ischemic stroke, 100
Islets of Langerhans, 26

J

Juvenile-onset diabetes. *See* Type 1 diabetes

K

Ketogenic diets, 76, 97
   cholesterol and, 86–89
Ketone bodies, 68
Ketosis, 97
Kidneys
   damage, 94
   health, 102–103

L

Lactose, 54, 66
Landmark clinical trials, 104
Legacy effect, 107, 109–110
Levemir, 305
Lifestyle changes, 7, 20, 37, 114, 166, 232
   defined, 15
   dietary habits, 15
   legacy effect of, 109–110
   physical activity, 15
Lifestyle journal, 179–182, 183t, 211
Linagliptin (Tradjenta), 298
Lipase, 30
Lipotoxicity, 29, 31
Liraglutide (Victoza), 300
Liver, 21
   detrimental changes, 78
   functions of, 21
   glycogen, 68
   insulin resistance, 57

muscle cells and, 23, 27
Lixisenatide (Adlyxin), 300
Lobeglitazone (Duvie), 302
Look AHEAD trial, 108
Low-carbohydrate diet, 46, 76
Low-density lipoprotein (LDL) cholesterol, 85
Luseogliflozin (Lusefi), 301
Lymphatic system, 27

M
Macular oedema, 101
Marine omega-3, 79
Maturity-Onset Diabetes of the Young (MODY), 38
Meal planning, 175, 179–229, 284–290
Meal sequencing, 213–214
Medications, 8–9, 47
  before exercise, 245
  GLP1/GIP agonists, 46
  glucose-lowering, 107
Meditation, 265–266
Mediterranean diet, 46, 81, 88, 108–109, 198, 213, 224
Metabolic memory, 107
Metformin (biguanide), 297
Microalbuminuria, 106
Microbiota, 158–159
Mifflin–St. Jeor formula, 198
Miglitol (Glyset), 300
Milk, 50
  carbohydrates, 66–67
  products, 54
Mindful eating, 124
  after eating, 137
  appetite, 130–131
  before eating, 136–137
  beginner's mind, 129–130
  defined, 126
  emotional eating, 137
  food emotion journal, 138t–139t
  fullness, 131–132
  hunger, 130
  hunger-fullness scale, 133t–134t
  hunger fullness tracker log, 134–135, 135t–136t
  mindfulness, 125–126
  raisin meditation, 127–129
  satiety, 131–132
Mindfulness, 125–126
Mindfulness-Based Stress Reduction (MBSR) program, 126
Minimally processed foods, 147
Mitochondrial function, 236
MODY. *See* Maturity-Onset Diabetes of the Young (MODY)
Monogenic diabetes syndromes, 38
Monosaccharides, 21, 52
Monotherapy, 297
Monounsaturated fatty acids (MUFA), 79, 224
Motivation, 114–117
Mounjaro (Tirzepatid), 300
MUFA. *See* Monounsaturated fatty acids (MUFA)
Multiple daily injections (MDI), 279

N
National Institute for Health and Care Excellence, 208
Neonatal Diabetes, 38
Nephropathy, 10
Nerves, 91. *See also* Neuropathy
  damage, 102
  peripheral, 102
Neuropathy, 10, 105
  autonomic, 102
  peripheral, 102
Neuroplasticity, 125
Neutral Protamine Hagedorn (NPH) insulin, 306

Night-time hypoglycaemia, 250
Non-insulin-dependent diabetes. *See* Type 2 diabetes
Non-sulfonylureas, 302
NOVA food classification system, 147
Novolin N, 305–306
Nurse's Health Study, 81
Nutrition Facts label, 82

O
Obesity, 14, 32–33
Obstructive sleep apnea, 254–255
OGTT. *See* Oral glucose tolerance test (OGTT)
Oligosaccharides, 54
Omega-3-fatty acids, 79–80, 215
Omega-6 fatty acids, 80
Oral glucose tolerance test (OGTT), 42
Oral Semaglutide (Rybelsus), 300

P
Packaged foods, 13–14, 192
Paleo diet, 76
Pancreas, 26, 28
Pancreatitis, 38
Peripheral neuropathy, 102
Peripheral vascular disease, 101
PERMA, 262–263
Physical activity, 15, 32, 214, 233–234
  blood glucose, 235
  type 2 diabetes, 36
Physical inactivity, 233
Phytonutrients, 218–219
Pilates, 244
Pioglitazone (Pioglit, Actos), 302
Plate pattern, 192
  fibre, 193–194
  right combination, 193
  right portions (quantity), 198–201, 199t–201t
  right proportion, 194, 194f–196f
  rule of 1:2 (grains: vegetables), 197–198
Polycystic ovary syndrome (PCOS), 1, 297
Polydipsia, 39
Polyphagia, 39
Polyphenols, 222
Polysaccharides, 21, 52, 54
Polyunsaturated fatty acids (PUFA), 79, 81
Polyuria, 39
Portion control, 210–212
Positive psychology, 262–263
Post-meal blood glucose, 209–210
Post-meal peak, 212
Post-meal physical exercise, 214
Prebiotics, 222
Prediabetes, 1–2, 113
  defined, 33
  diagnosis of, 6
PREDIMED study, 108–109
Pregnancy
  diabetes during, 2
  gestational diabetes mellitus, 36–37
  weight loss, 45
Pre-meal blood glucose, 184, 208
Premixed insulins, 305–306
Processed culinary ingredients, 147–148
Processed foods, 13, 59, 82, 146–148. *See also* Ultra-processed foods
Prostaglandins, 215
Proteins, 193, 213
PUFA. *See* Polyunsaturated fatty acids (PUFA)

R
Raisin meditation, defined, 127
Random plasma glucose test, 42
Real food, 13–14, 144–146, 166–167
  common barriers and empowerment, 170t
  culinary medicine, 169
  home cooking, 168
  identify and choose, 13
  preparation, 171
  storing, 172
Recipes, 291
  cauliflower rice topped with dal, 294–295
  chicken salad sandwich, 292–293
  date with oats, 296
  spicy sprout salad, 295–296
  sweet potato bake, 294
  vibrant vegetable frittata, 291–292
  zesty rice pilaf, 293
Refined carbohydrates
  examples of, 57
  excessive consumption of, 57
Refined grains, 58–60, 59f
Relapse, 227–229
Retinopathy, 101
Rosiglitazone (Avandia), 302
Roux-en-Y gastric bypass (RYGB), 46
Rule of 1:2 (grains: vegetables), 197–198

S
Satiety, 131–132
Saturated fats, 75–78
  excessive, consuming, 84–86
  high-fat diets, 76
  insulin resistance, 78
Saxagliptin (Onglyza), 298

Saxenda (liraglutide), 300
Self-monitoring of blood glucose (SMBG), 181
Semaglutide (Ozempic), 300
SGLT 2 inhibitors, 301
Short-chain fatty acids (SCFA), 67, 70
Simple carbohydrates, 53–57. *See also* Refined carbohydrates
  fruits and vegetables, 54
  milk and milk products, 54
  processed foods, 54
  sources of, 96
Sitagliptin (Januvia), 298
Skin problems, 103
Sleep disturbances
  inadequate, 254
  insomnia, 254
  obstructive sleep apnea, 254–255
Sleep hygiene, 255–257
Sleeping patterns, 214–215
Smart insulin pens, 278–279
Smart watches, 276–277
SMBG. *See* Self-monitoring of blood glucose (SMBG)
Smoking, 93
Strength training (resistance training), 239
Stress, 257
  chronic, 258, 267
  cognitive behavioural therapy, 260–262
  coping with, 260–266
  diabetes and, 259–260
  exercise, 265
  food and, 264–265
  management, 15–16
  meditation, 265–266
  positive psychology, 262–263
  self-help skills to, 264
  self-management techniques, 260–266

social interactions, 266
Stroke
   haemorrhagic, 100
   ischemic, 100
Sulfonylureas, 204, 302
Superfoods, 215–225

T

Talk test, 240
Tea, 219–221
Technology, 16–17, 269
   blood glucose
      continuous glucose monitoring, 271–273
      glucometers, 270–271
   diabetes
      apps, 274–275
      fitness trackers, 275–276
      insulin pump therapy, 279–281
      smart insulin pens, 278–279
      smart watches, 276–277
Thiazolidinediones (TZDs), 302
TIA. *See* Transient ischemic attack (TIA)
Tooth infections, 103
Trans fats, 81–82
Transient ischemic attack (TIA), 100
Triglycerides, 84
Triple therapy, 303
Troglitazone (Rezulin), 302
Type 1 diabetes, 11, 37–38
   diabetic ketoacidosis, 97
   risk factors for, 41
   symptoms of, 40
   warning signs of, 40
Type 2 diabetes, 5, 11, 14, 19, 35–36, 44, 87, 106
   chia seeds, 217
   circadian rhythms, 253–254
   coffee, 220
   diagnosis of, 36
   fat accumulation, 48
   genetic predisposition, 31
   glycemic load, 73
   injectables for, 303
   insomnia symptoms, 16
   insulin resistance, 19, 31
   mitochondrial dysfunction, 236
   natural history of, 35f
   obesity and, 32
   physical activity, 32
   poor sleeping habits, 16
   refined carbohydrates, 57
   remission, 45
   risk factors for, 41
   saturated fat, 76
   ultra-processed foods, 153
   weight loss, 32

U

Ulceration, 101
Ultra-processed foods, 82, 147
   accessibility and intake of, 152
   blood glucose levels, 155–157
   cancer, 168
   cardiovascular disease, 168
   choosing, 164–166
   daily intake of, 153
   defined, 148
   diabetes, 154
   feeling of hunger, 157–158
   food, craving for, 157–158
   gut health and, 158–161
   heart problems, 153
   inflammation and, 161–162
   insulin resistance, 155–157
   obesity, 168
   overeating, 163
   switching options, 165t

Index

United Kingdom Prospective Diabetes Study (UKPDS), 105–106
United States Department of Agriculture (USDA), 73, 83t
Unrefined carbohydrates, 57–58
Unsaturated fats, 78–79

V

Vegetables, 65–66, 150t, 193–194, 197–198, 222
Very-low-density lipoprotein (VLDL), 85
Vildagliptin (Galvus), 298
Vinegar, post-meal glycaemia, 213
Vitamins, 222

W

Wegovy (semaglutide), 300
Weight gain, 1, 6, 8, 23, 223
  during pregnancy, 37
  insulin resistance, 44
Weight loss, 20, 32, 45
  bariatric surgery, 46
  ketogenic diets, 86
  low-carbohydrate diet, 46
  Mediterranean diet, 46
  prediabetes, 34
  SGLT 2 inhibitors, 301
  unintentional, 39–40
White tea, 220
Whole grains, 58, 69
  consumption of, 60
  fibre and nutrients, 60
  glycemic index, 71
  research, 60–62
  structure of, 59f

www.ingramcontent.com/pod-product-compliance
Lightning Source LLC
LaVergne TN
LVHW091621070526
838199LV00044B/881